D0033759

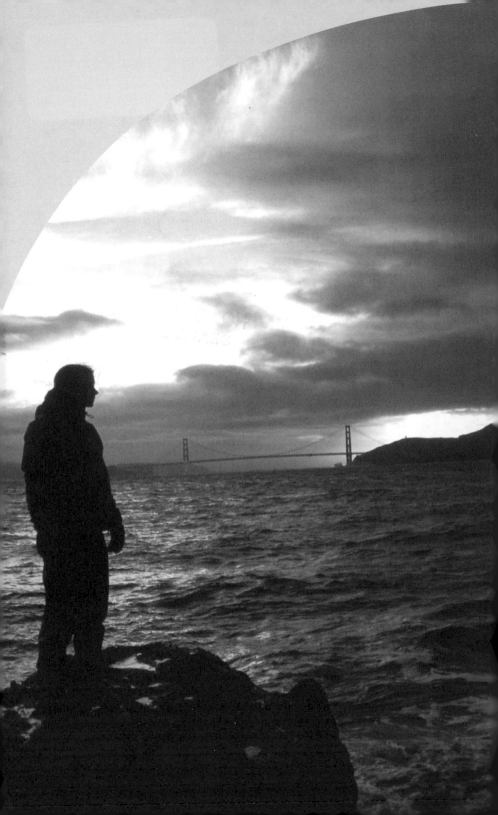

ONE NIGHT WILDERNESS
San Francisco Bay Area

Quick & convenient backpacking trips
within two hours of San Francisco

Matt Heid

 WILDERNESS PRESS ... *on the trail since 1967*

One Night Wilderness: San Francisco Bay Area:
Quick & convenient backpacking trips within two hours of San Francisco

1st EDITION 2011

Copyright © 2011 by Matt Heid
Front cover photo copyright © 2011 by Matt Heid
Interior photos, except where noted, by the author
Maps: Matt Heid and Scott McGrew
Cover design: Larry B. Van Dyke
Interior design: Lisa Pletka
Editor: Laura Shauger

ISBN 978-0-89997-623-5

Manufactured in the United States of America

Published by: Wilderness Press
                Keen Communications
                PO Box 43673
                Birmingham, AL 35243
                (800) 443-7227
                info@wildernesspress.com
                www.wildernesspress.com

Visit our website for a complete listing of our books and for ordering information.
Distributed by Publishers Group West

Cover photo: Above Tennessee Valley, Marin Headlands

Frontispiece: Perles Beach, Angel Island

SAFETY NOTICE: Although Wilderness Press and the author have made every attempt to ensure that the information in this book is accurate at press time, they are not responsible for any loss, damage, injury, or inconvenience that may occur to anyone while using this book. You are responsible for your own safety and health while in the wilderness. The fact that a trail is described in this book does not mean that it will be safe for you. Be aware that trail conditions can change from day to day. Always check local conditions, know your own limitations, and consult a map.

To Kieran
May you always love and protect Nature

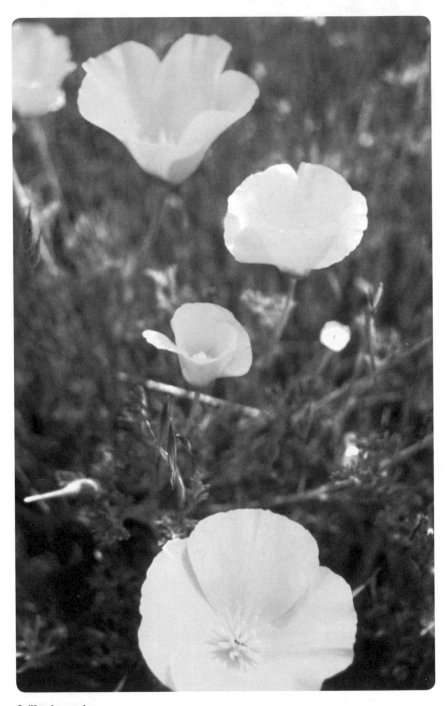

California poppies

Acknowledgments

Thanks go first to the innumerable rangers and park volunteers who aided in this book's research. Thank you for being the caring stewards of our parklands. I would particularly like to thank all of the employees of California State Parks, who have been forced to do more and more with less and less as the state grapples with its never-ending budget issues. Your dedication is appreciated by all who visit. Special thanks to Ted Jackson of Big Basin Redwoods State Park and John Verhoeven of Henry W. Coe State Park for their extensive assistance in providing the most up-to-date information for this book.

My deepest gratitude goes to all of you who have supported me over the years. To Gretchen, love of my life, for putting up with my dedication to this project. To my wonderful brother, who made possible an unforgettable journey on Tomales Bay, and to Analise for her constant encouragement to spend more time in California. To Dad and Joann, for always being there, including a bell-ringing tour of Angel Island. To Mom and Sid for your never-ending enthusiasm, love, and support of my passions. To Chuck Kapelke for taking the Mission Peak challenge. To Ben Hart for helping me fully enjoy the southern backcountry of Henry Coe. To the Ela family for their endless support. Finally, to my grandfather Albert Beck, for a lifetime of inspiration. May we all enjoy as many long, healthy, and happy years as you.

Thank you to my editor Laura Shauger, whose keen eye and steadfast hand helped guide this book to shining fruition. To Roslyn Bullas, for valiantly helming Wilderness Press and encouraging me to take on this project in the first place. To Molly Merkle and the staff at Keen Communications for accommodating this book during a time of challenging transition.

And to everybody, I say: Get out, have fun, and Hooray for Northern California!

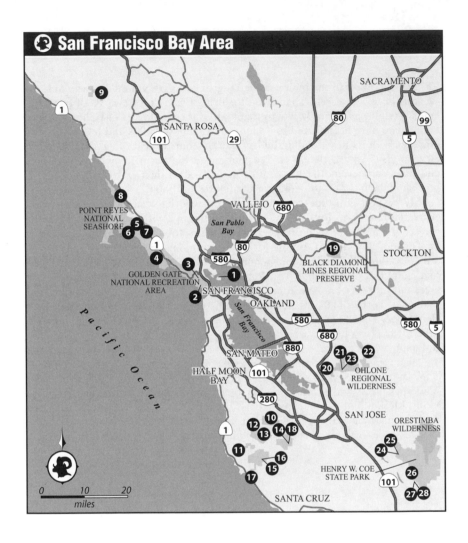

San Francisco Bay Area

SACRAMENTO

9

1

SANTA ROSA

101   29

80

99

5

8

POINT REYES
NATIONAL
SEASHORE   5
6   7
1

VALLEJO   680

San Pablo
Bay

4

80

3   580

19

BLACK DIAMOND
MINES REGIONAL
PRESERVE

STOCKTON

GOLDEN GATE
NATIONAL RECREATION
AREA   2

1

SAN FRANCISCO

OAKLAND

San Francisco
Bay

580

680

580

5

880

SAN MATEO

HALF MOON
BAY   101

21
23   22
20

OHLONE
REGIONAL
WILDERNESS

280

10

1   12   13   14   18

16

11

15

17

SAN JOSE

ORESTIMBA
WILDERNESS

25
24

HENRY W. COE
STATE PARK   101

26

27   28

SANTA CRUZ

Pacific Ocean

0   10   20
miles

Contents

Preface

Hundreds of parks, preserves, and protected open spaces infuse the San Francisco Bay Area with a world of unparalleled natural wonder. Straddling a remarkable range of geographic and ecological diversity, it provides avenues for adventure in all terrains, seasons, and environments. An overnight journey deepens this outdoor experience.

These 28 trips detail the best overnight backcountry opportunities in the greater Bay Area, from the deep valleys of the Coast Range to the old-growth redwoods of the Santa Cruz Mountains, from the shores of Point Reyes National Seashore to the remote corners of the Diablo Range in Henry Coe State Park. All of them are accessible within a two-hour drive from any point in the Bay Area.

Discovering all of these adventures on your own would be a formidable challenge. Nearly a dozen different governing agencies manage the parks of the Bay Area. Regulations, sources of information, and reservation systems vary widely by park district. The proximity of millions of people means that reservations are required for many destinations. Unraveling this complicated milieu on your own can be difficult and frustrating.

This book is the answer—a comprehensive guide to the best backpacking adventures in the San Francisco Bay Area. Within these pages you'll find detailed information on regulations, contact information, crowds, and reservations for every overnight destination—plus human history, natural history, trail descriptions, fun activities, maps, and lots of other good stuff. There is no better time to explore the magic of the Bay Area outdoors than right now. Have fun!

Point Reyes sunset

Summary of Featured Trips

EASY HIKES	SCENERY [1–10]	DIFFICULTY [1–10]	SOLITUDE [1–10]	MILES	ELEVEVATION GAIN	TRAIL USE
1 Angel Island State Park	9	1	1	2.6	+300'/–300'	kids
2 The Marin Headlands: Gerbode Valley Loop	8	3	3	7.3	+1,500'/–1,500'	kids
3 The Marin Headlands: Tennessee Valley	8	1	2	1.5	+250'/–250'	kids
4 Point Reyes: Wildcat Camp and Alamere Falls	7	4	3	11.0	+2,000'/–2,000'	
5 Point Reyes: Sky Camp to Palomarin	7	4	3	15.4	+2,300'/–2,980'	
10 Monte Bello Open Space Preserve Loop	5	2	5	5.0	+1,200'/–1,200'	kids
11 Butano State Park Loop	5	4	7	9.8	+2,100'/–2,100'	
12 Pescadero Creek County Park Loop	6	4	8	10.5	+1,500'/–1,500'	
13 Portola Redwoods State Park	5	3	4	5.0	+650'/–650'	
17 Big Basin Redwoods State Park: Inland from the Sea	7	4	4	2.0	+170'/–170'	kids

MODERATE HIKES	SCENERY [1–10]	DIFFICULTY [1–10]	SOLITUDE [1–10]	MILES	ELEVEVATION GAIN	TRAIL USE
6 Point Reyes: Coast Camp to Glen Camp Loop	6	5	3	16.9	+2,500'/–2,500'	
7 Point Reyes: Bear Valley Loop	6	5	3	15.8	+2,000'/–2,000'	
8 Point Reyes: Tomales Bay Boat-In Camping	8	5	8	4	Negligible	
9 Austin Creek State Recreation Area	7	6	8	6.4	+1,900'/–1,900'	
14 Castle Rock State Park Loop	8	5	5	5.2	+1,200'/–1,200'	

MODERATE HIKES	SCENERY [1–10]	DIFFICULTY [1–10]	SOLITUDE [1–10]	MILES	ELEVEVATION GAIN	TRAIL USE
15 Big Basin Redwoods State Park: Basin Trail Loop	7	5	7	11.6	+1,500'/1,500'	
16 Big Basin Redwoods State Park: Sunset Trail Camp Loop	10	6	1	10.0	+3,300'/–3,300'	
18 Skyline-to-the-Sea Trail	8	5	5	30	+2,500'/–5,100'	
19 Black Diamond Mines Regional Preserve	7	5	4	6.8	+1,700'/–1,700'	kids, dogs
20 Mission Peak Regional Preserve Loop	9	6	2	6.4	+2,000'/–2,000'	kids
21 Sunol Regional Wilderness: Sunol Backpack Camp Loop	8	6	7	5.9	+1,100'/–1,100'	kids
22 Del Valle Regional Park: Murietta Falls Loop	7	8	8	4.2	+1,600'/–1,600'	
28 Henry W. Coe State Park: Redfern Pond	7	6	8	7.6	+1,500'/–1,500'	kids

DIFFICULT HIKES	SCENERY [1–10]	DIFFICULTY [1–10]	SOLITUDE [1–10]	MILES	ELEVEVATION GAIN	TRAIL USE
23 The Ohlone Trail	10	8	9	28.2	+8,500'/–8,150'	
24 Henry W. Coe State Park: The Western Zone Loop	7	7	5	12.1	+2,500'/–2,500'	
25 Henry W. Coe State Park: Mississippi Lake and Beyond	7	10	10	24 – 50+	+6,000'/–6,000'	
26 Henry W. Coe State Park: Coit Lake and Vicinity	7	7	8	12.4	+3,800'/–3,800'	
27 Henry W. Coe State Park: Wilson Peak and Vicinity Loop	7	7	9	9.4	+2,500'/–2,500'	

Trips by Theme

GOOD FOR DOGS

LAKES AND PONDS

CREEKS AND RIVERS

FISHING

BOATING

GEOLOGY

REDWOOD FOREST

LESSER-TRAVELED DESTINATIONS

ACCESSIBLE BY PUBLIC TRANSPORTATION

3-5 DAY BACKPACKING TRIPS

EPIC VIEWS

AUTHOR'S FAVORITES

ONE NIGHT WILDERNESS

San Francisco Bay Area

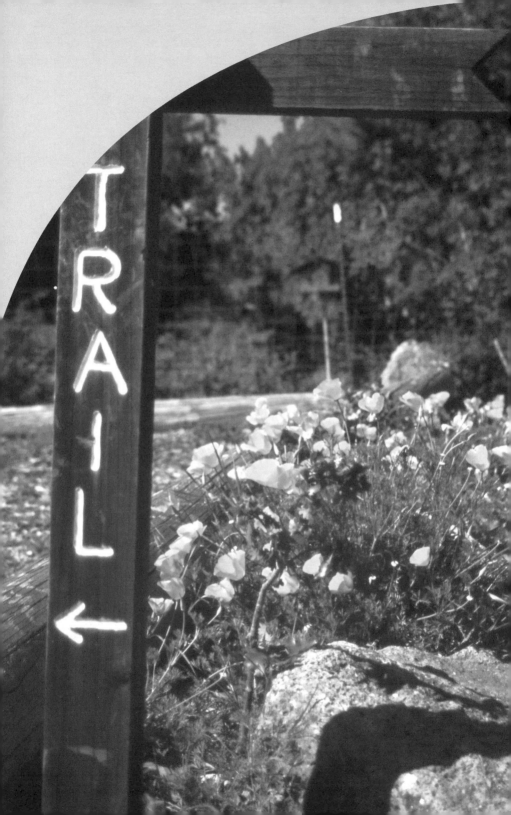

Introduction

How to Use This Book

This book divides the Bay Area into three geographic regions: the North Bay, Santa Cruz Mountains, and East of the Bay. Trips are listed in separate sections in that regional order. Each trip uses a standard format, described in greater detail below.

To prepare for your adventure, first read "Safety, Gear, and the Wilderness Ethic" (see page 4). Those unfamiliar with the outdoor world of the Bay Area or unsure about where to visit should consult "Where Should I Go?" (see page 12). For those looking for a specific feature, trips are grouped by theme after the Table of Contents (see page xiv). Otherwise simply flip through the pages and evaluate each adventure based on the standard information provided.

With the exception of Henry W. Coe State Park, all backpacking trips in the Bay Area require spending the night at a designated trail camp. The managing agency charges a fee for their use; most parks also require advance reservations. (Stiff fines are levied on those caught camping outside of designated areas.) Many trail camps offer amenities like picnic tables, food lockers, pit toilets, potable water, and obvious tent sites. Stoves are allowed at all trail camps; *campfires are prohibited almost everywhere. Dogs are prohibited on every backpacking trip in the Bay Area with the exception of Black Diamond Mines Regional Preserve.*

Trips are described using a standard, easily understood template. From top to bottom, the template is divided into four parts: Header, Planning Information, Hike Description, and Giving Back.

Header

TITLE Usually the park containing the hike, or a commonly used name for the hike (e.g., Skyline-to-the-Sea, see page 116).

RATINGS Below the title are numerical ratings (1 to 10) of three elements crucial to trip selection: scenery, difficulty, and solitude. The *scenery* rating is my subjective take on the trip's overall scenic qualities. All of the trips offer excellent scenery; some are just nicer than others. Trips rated 9 or 10 in this category offer particularly exceptional views or unique natural features found nowhere else.

The *difficulty* rating refers to the amount of effort and fitness required to complete the trip. Trips rated 1–3 travel on wide, easy trails over mostly level terrain; higher numbers correspond to greater distances. Trips rated 4–7 involve increasing amounts of distance and elevation change, ranging roughly from 1,000 to 2,000 feet per day. Trips rated 8–10 are strenuous adventures involving considerable and constant elevation gain of 2,000 to 3,000 feet per day across steep terrain and sometimes faint trails. Route-finding and bushwhacking may be required.

Let the adventure begin.

The *solitude* rating is a measure of how many people you will likely encounter on the hike. On trips rated 1–3 expect to encounter dozens of people throughout your hike, regardless of when you come. Trail camps will usually be full or nearly full. Trips rated 4–7 travel in areas where you will likely see some people during the trip, but not so many that it feels like a crowded experience. Some trips in this range will feature sections largely devoid of people, while other portions will be noticeably more popular. Trips rated 8–10 provide the opportunity for you to experience long stretches without seeing another soul.

ROUND-TRIP DISTANCE The total mileage of the hike. Most hikes are loop trips that do not retrace their steps. For point-to-point hikes, the one-way distance is listed.

ELEVATION GAIN/LOSS The amount of climbing and descending on the hike, measured in vertical feet. It can be significantly greater than the difference between the hike's lowest and highest points.

RECOMMENDED MAP Greater safety and enjoyment come with detailed, comprehensive maps—especially on hikes that traverse multiple parks or venture into more remote areas. The best available map for each trip is listed here. The maps included in this book are for initial planning purposes. If you want to take a particular trip, I strongly encourage you to acquire the suggested commercial or park-supplied map. Note that many state park maps may be difficult to locate outside of the associated park visitor center.

BEST TIMES The ideal season(s) to undertake the hike. Note that many of the trips can be done outside of the times listed, but weather or crowds make them less appealing.

AGENCY The managing agency for the specific park(s) visited on the trip.

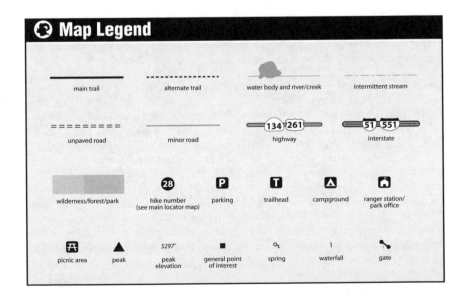

Basic contact information is included here.

PERMIT Basic information regarding the requisite backcountry or trail camp permit.

Planning Information

HIGHLIGHTS What makes the trip special, unique, and impossible to resist.

HIKE OVERVIEW A general description of the hike.

TRAIL CAMP(S) Detailed descriptions of trail camp(s), including location, natural surroundings, and facilities. This section includes detailed information about reservations and crowds, as well as regulations concerning capacity, maximum length of stay, and other restrictions.

GETTING THERE Gives concise driving directions to the trailhead. This book assumes you have a basic highway map of the Bay Area. If public transportation is available to the park, it is also listed here.

Hike Description

A detailed narrative of the hike itself. Parenthetical notations such as (3849') indicate elevation in feet. Parenthetical notations such as (3.2/1450') are included in the text at all trail junctions and important landmarks. The first number represents the total distance traveled from the trailhead in miles, the second identifies the location's elevation in feet.

Giving Back

A list of nonprofit groups that support the relevant parks through volunteer work or financial aid. Contact information is provided. Here is your chance to give something back to the natural world of the Bay Area so that others may enjoy the experience as you did.

Beating the Crowds

More than 7 million people live in the 10 greater Bay Area counties (Alameda, Contra Costa, Marin, Napa, San Francisco, San Mateo, Santa Clara, Santa Cruz, Solano, and Sonoma). Most of this dense collection of humanity exists around the common American schedule of busy weekdays, recreational weekends, and summer vacation. For the nearby and easily accessible parks of the Bay Area, this means that weekends are significantly—often exponentially—busier than weekdays. The crowd contrast between a weekday and weekend can be startling, with solitude one day and human torrents the next.

Summer is by far the busiest season. Most parks are busy on weekdays and absolutely packed on weekends and holidays from Memorial Day through Labor Day. Weekend crowds reduce as fall fades into winter and slowly increase once again as the rainy season tapers off in spring. Expect some full weekends for popular backpacking destinations in April, May, and October, but weekdays will be quiet everywhere from September through May. Overnight use is slight during the magical winter months from November through March.

Park usage varies widely. Parks in Marin County are visited considerably more than those in any other region in the Bay Area because of their scenic beauty, large contiguous acreage, and easy accessibility from much of the Bay Area. Weekends are particularly manic. Parks in the Santa Cruz Mountains and

East of the Bay are lesser visited and better for finding peace and quiet. Note that a few trail camps are first-come, first-served year-round—perfect for last-minute trips. These destinations, as well as those more lightly traveled, are listed in Trips by Theme (see page xiv).

Safety, Gear, and the Wilderness Ethic

Safety

Venturing into the outdoors entails a degree of risk. Preparation, knowledge, and awareness help mitigate that risk. The following section outlines the common hazards encountered in the Bay Area outdoors and discusses how to approach them.

Plant Hazards

POISON OAK If you recognize only one plant in California, it better be this one. Poison oak grows throughout the Bay Area and is particularly abundant in oak woodland and coastal scrub environments. A low-lying shrub or bush, its glossy, oaklike leaves grow in clusters of three and turn bright red in the fall before dropping off in the winter. Both the leaves and stems contain an oil (urushiol) that causes a strong allergic reaction in most people, creating a maddening and long-lived itchy rash where the oil contacts the skin. Wash thoroughly with soap within a few hours of exposure and clean clothing that may have come into contact with the plant. Residual oil on pants and dogs are prime rash culprits.

STINGING NETTLE This plant causes an unpleasant stinging sensation when any part of it comes into contact with your skin. It is common along the

coast, especially in Point Reyes National Seashore. Typically one to two feet tall, it can be recognized by its spiny leaves and the tiny stinging hairs that cover all parts of the plant. If it appears along a particular trail, I mention it in the hike description.

Wildlife Hazards

RATTLESNAKES Common throughout the eastern Bay Area, these venomous creatures like to bask on hot rocks in the sun and typically begin to emerge from winter hibernation as temperatures warm in spring. They usually flee at the first sight of people and will only attack if threatened. Be wary when hiking off-trail, and don't put your hands where you can't see them when scrambling on rocky slopes. Rattlesnake bites are rarely fatal. If you are bitten, the goal is to reduce the rate at which the poison circulates through your body—try to remain calm, keep the bite site below the level of your heart, remove any constricting items (rings, watches, etc.) from the soon-to-be swollen extremity, and do not apply ice or chemical cold to the bite as this can cause further damage to the surrounding tissue. Seek medical attention as quickly as possible.

TICKS These parasites love brushy areas and are common throughout the Bay Area, especially during the rainy season. Always perform regular body checks when hiking through tick country. If you find a tick attached to you, do not try to pull it out with your fingers or to pinch the body; doing so can increase the risk of infection. Using an appropriate tool, gently pull the tick out by lifting upward from the base of the body where it is attached to your skin. Pull straight out until the tick releases, and do not twist or jerk as this may break the mouthparts off under your skin. Tweezers work for this operation, though not as well as the many lightweight and inexpensive tick removal tools available.

Ticks are known for transmitting Lyme disease, but only one of the 48 tick species in California is capable of transmitting it—the diminutive western black-legged tick—and chances are low for exposure. Even if you are bitten, an infected tick must be attached for a minimum of six hours in order to transmit the disease. Caused by a spirochete, Lyme disease can be life-threatening if not diagnosed in its early phases. Common early symptoms include fatigue, chills and fever, headache, muscle and joint pain, swollen lymph nodes, and a blotchy skin rash that clears centrally to produce a characteristic ring shape 3–30 days after exposure. If you fear that you have been exposed to Lyme disease, consult a doctor immediately.

GIARDIA *Giardia lamblia* is a microscopic organism occasionally found in backcountry water sources. Existing as a dormant cyst while in the water, it develops in the gastrointestinal tract upon consumption and can cause diarrhea, excessive flatulence, foul-smelling excrement, nausea, fatigue, and abdominal cramps. The risk of contraction is low in the Bay Area's backcountry waterways, but the potential consequences are worth preventing. All water taken from the backcountry should be purified with a filter, a chemical treatment, or by boiling it for three minutes.

RACCOONS, SKUNKS, AND FOXES While not a threat to humans, these nocturnal scavengers have learned that campgrounds and trail camps are prime locations for free meals. They are a major hazard for food supplies.

Never leave your food unattended and always store it somewhere safe at night. Food lockers are provided at most trail camps; otherwise hang it from a nearby tree. Bringing food into the tent with you is *never* a good idea.

MOUNTAIN LIONS These large felines roam throughout much of the Bay Area backcountry but are rarely seen and pose minimal threat. If you do encounter an aggressive mountain lion, make yourself look as large as possible and do not run away. If you have children with you, pick them up.

BEARS Once common throughout the Bay Area, grizzly and black bears were eliminated from the region in the 1800s by unregulated hunting. In recent years, however, there have been several confirmed black bear sightings in Point Reyes National Seashore and around Mount Tamalpais. Bear populations may be slowly expanding back into former Bay Area habitat, though the odds of actually encountering one are extremely low.

Physical Dangers

HYPOTHERMIA This life-threatening condition occurs when the body is unable to stay adequately warm and its core temperature begins to drop. Initial symptoms include uncontrollable shivering, mental confusion, slurred speech, and weakness. Cold, wet weather poses the greatest hazard as wet clothes conduct heat away from the body much faster than dry layers. Fatigue reduces your body's ability to produce its own heat, and wind poses an increased risk as it can quickly strip away warmth. In the Bay Area, the cold, damp months of winter create prime hypothermic conditions.

Immediate treatment is critical. Raise the body's core temperature as quickly as possible. Get out of the wind, take off wet clothes, drink warm beverages, eat simple energy foods, and take shelter in a warm tent or sleeping bag. Do not drink alcohol as this dilates the blood vessels and causes increased heat loss.

HEATSTROKE The opposite of hypothermia, heatstroke occurs when the body is unable to control its internal temperature and overheats. Usually brought on by excessive exposure to the sun and accompanying dehydration, symptoms include cramping, headache, and mental confusion. Treatment entails rapid, aggressive cooling of the body through whatever means available—cooling the head and torso is most important. Stay hydrated and have some type of sun protection for your head if you expect to travel along a hot, exposed section of trail. Parks located east of the Bay have plenty of scorching heat and shadeless terrain during the summer months, posing the region's greatest risk for heatstroke.

SUNBURN The Bay Area sun can fry you quickly, even if the sky is overcast with light fog or clouds. Always wear sunscreen of sufficiently high SPF, and don a hat or visor to shield your face from the sun. Don't forget to protect your ears and lips! Make sure your sunscreen protects from both UVB rays, which cause sunburn (this is what SPF measures), and UVA, which causes premature aging of the skin and wrinkles. Read sunscreen labels closely to ensure they also block UVA—many do not.

THE PACIFIC OCEAN The waters of the Pacific are frigid (temperature in the 50s year-round), swirling with strong currents, and ripping with undertows that can quickly suck the unwary out to sea. Rogue waves can occur at any time, sweeping the unsuspecting from seemingly safe rocks and beaches—but are especially likely during times of large swell. Unless you are confident in your swimming ability and knowledge of the ocean, don't tempt fate by going into the water.

Hiking Safety

LEAVE AN ITINERARY Always tell somebody where you are hiking and when you expect to return. Friends, family, rangers, and visitor centers are all valuable resources that can save you from a backcountry disaster if you fail to reappear on time.

KNOW YOUR LIMITS Don't undertake a hike that exceeds your physical fitness or outdoor abilities.

AVOID HIKING ALONE A hiking partner can provide the margin between life and death in the event of a serious backcountry mishap.

BRING THE RIGHT GEAR Packing the proper equipment, especially survival and first-aid supplies, increases your margin of safety.

Gear

Survival Essentials

Always have with you:

WATER Carry at least one liter of water (preferably two), drink frequently, and have some means of purifying backcountry sources (chemical treatment or filter).

FIRE AND LIGHT Bring waterproof matches and quick-lighting tinder for an emergency fire and a headlamp or flashlight for the night.

FIRST-AID KIT At minimum a first-aid kit should include an over-the-counter painkiller/swelling reducer (ibuprofen is always good); a two- to four-inch-wide elastic (ACE) bandage for wrapping sprained ankles, knees, and other joints; and the basics for treating a bleeding wound: antibiotic ointment, sterile gauze, small bandages, medical tape, and large band-aids. Prepackaged kits are readily available.

MAP AND COMPASS These two essentials can help you find your way home. Even the simplest compass is useful.

KNIFE A good knife can be invaluable in the event of a disaster. Pocketknives and all-in-one tools have many other useful features as well.

EXTRA CLOTHES AND FOOD Warm clothing can be critical in the event of an unexpectedly cold or wet night. A few extra energy bars can make a huge difference in your morale and energy level if you are out longer than expected.

OTHER GOOD IDEAS A whistle is a powerful distress signal and can save your life if you become immobilized. Sunscreen and sunglasses protect you from blazing sun.

For Your Feet

Your feet are your most important piece of gear. Keep them happy, and you will be even more so. Appreciate them. Care for them.

FOOTWEAR The appropriate hiking footwear provides stability and support for your feet and ankles while protecting them from the abuses of the environment. Most trails in the Bay Area present little in the way of rough or uneven terrain. A pair of lightweight hiking boots or trail running shoes is generally adequate for most hikes, though hikers with weak ankles may want to opt for heavier, mid-weight hiking boots.

When selecting footwear, keep in mind that the most important feature is a good fit—your toes should not hit the front while going downhill, your heel should be locked in place inside the boot to prevent friction and blisters, and there should be minimal extra space around your foot (although you

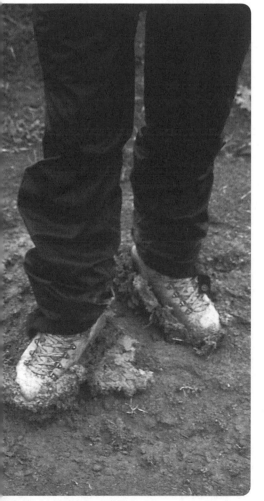

Winter mud walking at Black Diamond Mines Regional Preserve

should be able to wiggle your toes free-ly). When lacing them, leave the laces over the top of your foot (instep) loose but tie them tightly across the ankle to lock the heel down.

Stability over uneven ground is enhanced by a stiffer sole and higher ankle collar—good for those with weak ankles. All-leather boots last longer, have a good deal of natural water resistance, and will mold to your feet over time. Some boots have Gore-Tex or an equivalent waterproof-breathable layer and are excellent for wet winter hikes. Break in new boots before taking them on an extended hike to minimize the chances for blisters—simply wear them around as much as possible beforehand.

SOCKS After armpits, feet are the sweatiest part of the human body—and wet feet are much more prone to blisters. Good hiking socks wick moisture away from your skin and provide padding for your feet. Avoid cotton socks as these quickly saturate, stay wet inside your shoes, and take forever to dry. Many socks are a confusing mix of natural and synthetic fibers. Wool provides warmth and padding and, while it does absorb roughly 30 percent of its weight in water, effectively keeps your feet dry. If regular wool makes your feet itch, try softer merino wool. Nylon, polyester, acrylic, and polypropylene (also called olefin) are all synthetic fibers that absorb very little water, dry quickly, and add durability. Thin liner socks are worn underneath your principal socks and are designed to more effectively wick moisture away—good for really sweaty feet.

BLISTER KIT As everybody knows, blisters suck. They are almost always caused by friction from foot movement

(slippage) inside the shoe. Prevent blisters by buying properly fitting footwear, taking a minimum of one to two weeks to break them in, and wearing appropriate socks. If your heel is slipping and blistering, try tightening the laces across your ankle to keep the heel in place. If you notice a blister or hotspot developing, stop immediately and apply adhesive padding (such as moleskin) over the problem spot. Bring a lightweight pair of scissors to easily cut the moleskin.

Outdoor Clothing

The following information is useful for staying warm and dry in camp or on the trail.

FABRICS Cotton is a lousy fabric for outdoor activity and should be avoided. It absorbs water quickly and takes a long time to dry, leaving a cold, wet layer next to your skin and increasing the risk of hypothermia. Jeans are the worst. In hot, dry environments, however—such as those found east of the Bay during the summer months—cotton is useful as the water it retains helps keep you cool as it evaporates.

Polyester and nylon are two commonly used, and recommended, fibers in outdoor clothing. They dry almost instantly, wick moisture effectively, and are lighter weight than natural fibers. Fleece clothing (made from polyester) provides good insulation and will keep you warm even when wet. Synthetic materials melt quickly, however, if placed in contact with a heat source (campstove, fire, sparks, etc.). Wool is a good natural fiber for hiking. Despite the fact that it retains up to 30 percent of its weight in water, it still insulates when wet. A lightweight down vest or jacket adds considerable warmth for minimal bulk and weight, though must be kept dry—wet down loses all of its insulating ability.

RAINGEAR AND WINDGEAR There are three types of raingear and windgear available: waterproof and breathable, waterproof and nonbreathable, and water-resistant. Waterproof, breathable shells contain Gore-Tex or an equivalent material and effectively keep liquid water out while still allowing water vapor (i.e., your sweat) to pass through. They keep you more comfortable during heavy exertions in the rain (though you will still get damp from the inside) and are generally bulky and more expensive.

Waterproof, nonbreathable shells are typically made from coated nylon or a rubberlike material. They keep water out but hold all your sweat in. Seams must be taped for them to be completely waterproof. Although wearing these on a strenuous hike is a hot and sticky experience, they are cheap and often very lightweight.

Water-resistant shells are usually lightweight nylon windbreakers coated with a water-repellent chemical. The seams are *not* taped. They will often keep you dry for a short time but will quickly soak through in a heavy rain. All three are good in the wind. In the Bay Area, a lightweight windbreaker is all you need from May through October when rain is a rarity but coastal and inland breezes common. During winter months, however, fully waterproof raingear is recommended.

KEEPING YOUR HEAD AND NECK WARM The three most important parts of the body to insulate are the torso, neck, and head. Your body will strive to keep these a constant temperature at all times. Without any insulation, the heat coursing through your neck to your brain radiates out into space and is lost. Warmth that might have been directed to your extremities is instead spent replacing the heat lost from your head. A thin balaclava or warm hat and neck gaiter are small items, weigh almost nothing, and are more effective at keeping you warm than an extra jacket.

KEEPING YOUR HANDS WARM Hiking in cold and damp conditions (such as those found in a redwood forest) will often chill your hands unpleasantly. A lightweight pair of synthetic liner gloves will do wonders.

Backpacking Equipment

BACKPACK For most people, an overnight pack with 3,000 to 4,000 cubic inches of capacity is generally necessary, though ultralight hikers can get away with less. When shopping for a pack, keep in mind that the most important feature is a good fit. A properly fitting backpack allows you to carry the vast majority of weight on your hips and lower body, sparing the easily fatigued muscles of the shoulders and back.

When trying on packs, loosen the shoulder straps, position the waist belt so that the top of your hips (the bony iliac crest) is in the middle of the belt, attach and cinch the waist belt, and then tighten the shoulder straps. The waist belt should fit snugly around your hips, with no gaps. The shoulder straps should rise slightly off your shoulders before dipping back down to attach to the pack about an inch below your shoulders—weight should *not* rest on top of your shoulders, and you should be able to shrug them freely.

Most packs will have load stabilizer straps that attach to the pack behind your ears and lift the shoulder straps upward, off of your shoulders. A sternum strap links the two shoulder straps together across your chest and prevents them from slipping away from your body. Most packs are highly adjustable—a knowledgeable employee at an outdoor equipment shop can be invaluable in helping you achieve the proper fit.

Load your pack to keep its center of gravity as close to your middle and lower back as possible. Heaviest items should go against your back, and you should pack items from heaviest to lightest outward and upward. Do not place heavy items at or below the level of the hip belt—doing so precludes the ability to carry that weight on the lower body and is one of the main reasons packs feature sleeping bag compartments in that location.

SLEEPING BAG Nights are surprisingly cool year-round in the Bay Area. Freezing conditions are uncommon, but you should expect nighttime temperatures in the 50s most of the year with dips into the 40s and even 30s during the winter. For hikers who sleep cold, a bag rated to 20°F is recommended for all-purpose use; those who sleep warm should find a 30–35°F bag adequate.

Down sleeping bags offer the highest warmth-to-weight ratio, are incredibly compressible, and will easily last a decade or more without losing much of their loft. However, down loses all of its insulating ability when wet and takes forever to dry—a genuine concern during the rainy Bay Area winters. Synthetic-fill sleeping bags retain their insulating abilities even when wet and are cheaper, but the increased bulk and weight is a drawback. Synthetic-fill bags lose some of their loft and insulating ability after a few seasons of use.

SLEEPING PAD Sleeping pads offer vital comfort and insulation from the cold ground. Inflatable, foam-filled pads (such as Therm-a-Rest) are the most compact and comfortable to sleep on, but expensive and mildly time-consuming to inflate and deflate. Basic foam pads are lightweight, cheap, and virtually indestructible. Comfort makes the call.

TENT A lightweight, three-season tent is all that most Bay Area backpacking trips require; ultralight hikers can forgo a tent entirely during the dry months. Two-person backpacking tents average between four to five pounds and feature transparent, weight-saving mesh on the tent body. A rainfly that extends to the ground on all sides is critical for staying dry.

Leaks are typically caused by water seeping through unsealed seams and/or contact between a wet rainfly and the tent body. Seal any untaped seams that are directly exposed to the rain or to water running off the fly—pay close attention to the floor corners. Pitch the tent as tautly as possible to keep a wet and saggy rainfly away from the tent body.

Most trail camps in the Bay Area offer good shelter from the wind, though a few do not. Stability in wind is enhanced by pole intersections—the more poles and the more times they cross, the stronger the tent will be in blustery conditions. Placing a tarp between the tent floor and the ground will protect the floor from ground moisture, wear and tear, and will increase the lifespan of your tent. Most tents have an optional footprint that exactly matches the floor—a nice accessory.

COOKING EQUIPMENT A stove is necessary if you want hot food on the trail; *campfires are prohibited virtually everywhere in the Bay Area.* Two types of stoves are available. Canister stoves run on a butane and propane blend pressurized in a metal canister. Simply attach the stove burner to the canister, turn the knob, and light. Such stoves are simple, safe, cheap, and have an adjustable flame. Their safety and simmer-ability make them a good choice for Bay Area backpacking, though they do have some drawbacks. Canisters are usually available only at outdoor equipment stores, are difficult to recycle, do not work below freezing, and heat very slowly when less than a quarter full.

Liquid fuel stoves run on white gas contained in a self-pressurized tank or bottle. White gas is inexpensive, burns hot, is widely available around the world, and works in extremely cold conditions. You must work directly with liquid fuel to prime the stove, however, adding an element of danger. They're also prone to flaring up, often do not have an adjustable flame, and are more expensive. Liquid fuel stoves are a good choice for those interested in winter camping or international travel.

A simple two- to three-quart pot is all that most people need for backcountry cooking. Add a small frying pan if necessary. A black, or blackened, pot will absorb heat more quickly and increase fuel efficiency. A windscreen for the stove is helpful in breezy conditions. The only dish needed is a plate with upturned edges, which can double as a broad bowl—a Frisbee or gold pan works well. Don't forget the silverware! Lastly, an insulated mug is essential for enjoying hot drinks.

OTHER GOOD STUFF A length of nylon cord is useful for hanging food, stringing clotheslines, and guying out tents. A simple repair kit should include needle, thread, and duct tape. A plastic trowel is nice for digging crapholes. Insect repellent will keep the bugs away. A pair of sandals or running shoes for around camp are a great relief from hiking boots. A pen and waterproof notebook allow you to record outdoor epiphanies on the spot. Extra ziplock or garbage bags always come in handy. Compression stuff sacks will reduce the bulk of your sleeping bag and clothes by about a third.

FUN EQUIPMENT Make sure your camera is ready for outdoor abuse and keep it safe from dirt and moisture. A good protective camera bag costs much less than a new camera. A polarizing filter is good for taking outdoor pictures with lots of sky and water. Shady forests are challenging to photograph when the sun is out—wait for foggy or overcast days and carry a small tripod for shooting in the low-light conditions. An altimeter is a fun toy for tracking your progress and identifying your location. See more with binoculars. Play more with a hacky sack, Frisbee, cards, or other backcountry games.

The Wilderness Ethic

To preserve the Bay Area outdoors for future generations, follow some simple guidelines to leave no trace of your passage:

DO NOT SCAR THE LAND Do not cut switchbacks. Stay on the trail as much as possible. Leave rocks, plants, and other natural objects as you find them.

CAMPING Camp only at established sites. Do not dig ditches around your tent. Keep your camp clean and never leave food out. Confine activities to where vegetation is absent.

FIRES   Campfires, where allowed, should always be made in a fire ring. In the Bay Area, *wood collecting of any kind is prohibited.* Make sure your fire is completely out before leaving.

SANITATION   When nature calls, choose a spot at least 200 feet away from trails, water sources, and campsites. Dig a cathole at least six inches deep, make your deposit, and cover it with the soil you removed. Do not bury toilet paper.

WASHING   To wash yourself or your dishes, carry water 200 feet away from streams or lakes. Scatter strained dishwater. Avoid using soap if possible, otherwise use only small amounts of biodegradable soap.

GARBAGE   Carry out all garbage and burn only paper. Thoroughly inspect your site for trash and spilled food before leaving.

GROUP SIZE   Keep groups small to minimize impact.

ANIMALS   Do not feed wildlife. Observe only from a distance. If an animal changes its behavior because of your presence, you are too close. If you meet horse on the trail, move off the trail on the downhill side and stand still until the animal passes by.

NOISE   Be respectful of other wilderness users. Listen to the sounds of nature.

Where Should I Go?

Blessed with mild year-round weather and tremendous natural diversity, the Bay Area offers a wide variety of overnight outdoor adventures for every month of the year. To help you choose the perfect overnight adventure, the following sections describe the geography, weather, ecosystems, and governing agencies of the Bay Area outdoors. A Season-by-Season Playbook (see page 16) summarizes all three factors into a year-round cycle of Bay Area outdoor fun.

Bay Area Geography

The landscape of the Bay Area has been crushed by colliding tectonic plates, sliced by massive faults, and squeezed upward into a rumpled world of rolling hills, steep ridges, and deep valleys with an overall convoluted topography. For the purpose of this book, the region's unique geography is roughly grouped into three regions: the North Bay, Santa Cruz Mountains, and East of the Bay. A general overview of each region's geography and featured parks follows.

North Bay

The North Bay includes the region found north of the Golden Gate and is characterized by rugged topography and a wild coastline. A series of high ridges and peaks geographically isolates the western coastal areas from the population centers found closer to the Bay. Farther east, linear Sonoma and Napa valleys lie between mountainous ridges of volcanic rock. The region is remarkable for its large amount of easily accessible protected open space available for exploration—44 percent of Marin County is composed of parks, preserves, and other public land.

All of the backpacking opportunities, however, are found in the western regions closer to the coast, with Point Reyes National Seashore and the Marin Headlands the principal destinations. They are two of the most scenic, popular, and crowded parks in the Bay Area.

For a more remote experience, the book reaches as far north as Austin Creek State Recreation Area, a more distant destination tucked in the folds of the Coast Ranges near the Russian River.

Santa Cruz Mountains

The Santa Cruz Mountains extend south from Half Moon Bay to Santa Cruz and then west to the Santa Clara Valley south of San Jose. A rugged, ridge-lined landscape deeply incised by a multitude of creeks, the geography is largely defined by the axis of long, northwest-trending Skyline Ridge. Stretching more than 50 miles from near Gilroy to Highway 92 above Half Moon Bay, it rises some 3,000 feet and separates the developed Bay Area from the wild heart of these mountains. West of Skyline Ridge, a multitude of creeks and rivers tumble toward the ocean, the largest of which are (from north to south) Pescadero Creek, Waddell Creek, and the San Lorenzo River. Redwood forest characterizes most outdoor adventures in the region.

Most of the Santa Cruz Mountains and its protected parklands are located along the west side of Skyline Ridge. In the heart of the mountains lies a large complex of contiguous and interconnected parks centered around the Pescadero and Waddell creek drainages—Sam McDonald, Memorial, and Pescadero Creek county parks and Portola Redwoods, Butano, Castle Rock, and Big Basin Redwoods state parks. With the exception of Butano, all of these parks either border each other or are connected via a network of trails. With more than 10 backcountry trail camps in this complex, opportunities for overnight adventures among the redwoods are extensive. Experience the full diversity of the Santa Cruz Mountains on the Skyline-to-the Sea Trail, a 30-mile journey from Skyline Ridge to the Pacific Ocean.

East of the Bay

For the purposes of this book, East of the Bay includes the ecologically similar regions found east of San Francisco Bay and the Santa Clara Valley. A multitude of north-south trending ridges compose the hilly terrain found East of the Bay, offering little in the way of level ground. In the northern area, monolithic Mt. Diablo dominates; at 3,849 feet it towers over the surrounding landscape and overlooks the lower-lying Oakland and Berkeley Hills to the west. Farther south, the land is wrinkled into the tortured Diablo Range, a series of furrowed ridges and peaks rising 3,000 feet and higher.

Backpacking trips are largely confined to two destinations: Henry W. Coe State Park and the Ohlone Trail, which spans Mission Peak Regional Preserve, Sunol Regional Wilderness, Ohlone Regional Wilderness, and Del Valle Regional Park. Both offer opportunities to explore the Bay Area's deepest backcountry on extended multiday excursions, as well as on shorter, overnight trips. The only other backpacking option is Black Diamond Mines Regional Preserve, a place of rich history, woodlands, and wildlife in the eastern Mt. Diablo foothills.

Bay Area Geology

A long, long time ago, the western edge of North America was in the vicinity of today's Sierra Nevada foothills. Offshore, a massive tectonic plate was being slowly driven beneath the continent. Covered by the ocean for millions of years, the tectonic plate had accumulated deep layers of sand, mud, and microscopic sea creature skeletons on its rocky underwater surface. As the plate slid beneath prehistoric California, this collection of mud, sand, skeletons, and rocks was scraped off, scrambled in a deep offshore trench, and left a confused and jumbled mix that today has risen to form most of the San Francisco Bay Area landscape.

This jumble is known as the Franciscan Formation. Several common rock types are associated with it and regularly appear in campgrounds and on backpacking trips in the Bay Area. Chert formed from the accumulated silica-rich skeletons and is easily recognized by its obvious layering, resistance to erosion (often found in cliff faces and rock outcrops), sharp edges, and typical dark red coloration (although it can also appear a pale, translucent white or green). Sandstone is easily recognized by its brown color, rough surfaces, and tiny sand grains. Shale is hardened, compressed mud and is identified by its microscopic grains, a gray-black coloration, and its tendency to fracture in a rectangular fashion.

Greenstone, or pillow basalt, comes from the deep rocks of the sea floor and is formed as molten rock is forced to the underwater surface from deep within the earth. Also highly resistant to erosion, it appears frequently in cliffs and on rocky shores and is identified by its green color on freshly broken faces, lack of layering, and by the one- to three-foot bulbous masses (the "pillows") that are often identified in exposures. Serpentine, California's state rock, comes from the bowels of the earth where rocks first solidify above molten material. Scraped off and jumbled near the surface, it reacts with groundwater to form a slippery, waxy green rock.

The region west of the San Andreas Fault tells a different geologic tale. Once upon a time, after the rock scramble described above, the San Andreas Fault was born somewhere in Southern California. Land west of the fault was ripped from its moorings and moved northward. Formed principally of the same granite that today sits in the southern Sierra Nevada, this migrant piece of California was buried beneath the sea on its journey north and blanketed with mud and sand. Today it has been pushed back above the surface to form the rugged hills found west of the fault—the western Santa Cruz Mountains and Point Reyes peninsula. While loosely consolidated sandstone and mudstone still cover most of the underlying granite, the unique salt-and-pepper color of granitic rock does appear in places.

Weather of the San Francisco Bay Area

The Bay Area is characterized by a Mediterranean climate. To put it simply: From November through April, it rains; from May through October, it doesn't. Snow is rare, temperatures are mild year-round, and outdoor excursions are possible in every month of the year.

Dry Season: May Through October

During this period, Bay Area weather is dominated by two things: sun and fog. It seldom rains, leaving most areas to bask in hot solar rays. Temperatures become increasingly warm farther inland, with readings in the 90s not uncommon for many regions east of the Bay. Meanwhile, over the cold Pacific Ocean, fog forms. Moisture contained in warm summer air condenses over the frigid waters into a ground-hugging cloud, which prevailing winds then push onshore.

What Drives the Weather

The Bay Area's weather patterns are determined primarily by a dominating influence known as the Pacific High. Wherever the sun most directly strikes the earth, air near the surface is warmed, loses pressure, and rises into the upper atmosphere. Closer to the chill of space, this heated column of air then cools as it moves toward the poles. As the temperature drops, the air increases in density and consequently sinks toward the surface to form a large area of high pressure.

From May through September, the sun most directly strikes the northern hemisphere, causing a large zone of high pressure to form over the North Pacific Ocean between roughly 35°N and 40°N latitude. Located at 38°N, the San Francisco Bay Area receives the effects of this Pacific High from May, when it first forms, through October, when its long-stabilized presence finally dissipates as the sun moves over the southern hemisphere. Forcing the eastward-flowing jet stream to the north, the Pacific High prevents storms brewed in the Gulf of Alaska from reaching California and creates the hot, dry days of the Bay Area summer. However, it also creates conditions perfect for the development of coastal fog and wind.

Air flows from areas of high pressure to regions of low pressure, which means that winds flow from the Pacific High toward the lower pressure zones found inland. Slightly twisted in direction by the Coriolis effect, these cool winds consequently strike Northern California's coast from the northwest for as long as the Pacific High is present. What's more, ocean surface water moves perpendicular to wind direction. As a result, warmer surface waters near land are pushed offshore by the prevailing winds, leaving a void that colder water from the ocean depths fill. With temperatures in the low 50s, this frigid water chills the air above it. Cold air holds less moisture than warm air, and thus upon contact with the cold ocean waters, the nicely heated summer air suddenly condenses into thick, soupy, chilly *fog*.

In October and November, as the sun strikes the earth farther down the southern hemisphere, the Pacific High dissipates. No longer impeded by the zone of high pressure, the jet stream flows over California and brings with it the storms of winter. From November through March, these storms regularly lash the Bay Area until, once again, the sun returns north to rebuild the Pacific High.

Flowing inland like an airborne river, the low-lying fog is typically blocked by the high ridges of the Santa Cruz Mountains and North Bay, but low fog gaps—such as the Golden Gate—allow it to penetrate deeper inland.

The farther inland, the more likely the fog will burn off by late morning or early afternoon. Meanwhile, coastal destinations can smother under fog for days on end, with brisk onshore winds blowing from the northwest. Fog is common throughout the summer, is at its thickest in July and August, and tapers off as September fades into October.

Haze, heat, and fog are common from May through August, and finding an ideal outdoor destination can be challenging. Shady redwood forest is always a good option during this period. The Indian summer months of September and October still bring bouts of fog and inland heat, but are also the months most likely to produce sunny, warm days perfect for exploring anywhere across the region. In the fall a dash of color can be seen along creeks in the yellow leaves of sycamores and bigleaf maples, heralding the return of the . . .

Rainy Season: November Through April

As the winter months approach, the jet stream flows south over Northern California and brings with it winter storms born in the Gulf of Alaska. Rain drenches the Bay Area as cold fronts regularly sweep through, becoming increasingly frequent as the winter months progress. Strong winds typically blow from the south as the fronts approach; a storm can drop several inches of rain in a day's time, making for extremely wet and windy outdoor conditions. While the higher elevations (2,000 feet or higher) around the Bay Area receive an occasional snow flurry in the winter months, it is a rare occurrence.

In a typical year, the first rogue storms arrive sometime in late October, increase in frequency during November and December, hit hardest in January and February (the wettest months), and start tapering off in March. April tends to be unpredictable; summerlike days (complete with coastal fog) are as likely as cold wintry storms.

The weather may be more challenging during the rainy season, but these are the glory months for outdoor adventure in the Bay Area. Warm sunny breaks regularly occur between storm fronts and can last for days, especially in the shoulder months of November and April. The wind and storms purge the air of smog and haze, leaving behind crystalline views. The first rains of the season pour life into a landscape that quickly flourishes green, exploding with wildflowers from late February until May. Winter waves along the coast become large and powerful, an impressive display of nature's power. Keep a close eye on the weather forecast and windows of sunny opportunity will always open, for now the entire Bay Area is empty and open for outdoor adventure.

A Season-by-Season Playbook

Winter (December–February)

Winter is a magical time. Slaked with moisture after months of dry weather, open landscapes blush a luminescent green. The air of the Bay Area is purged by wind and cleansed by rain, creating sparkling and far-reaching views. In the redwood forest, countless mushrooms explode as orange-bellied newts clamber across the eternally damp forest floor. Streams and waterfalls flow strong across the land, gushing at peak volume. The naked limbs of deciduous oaks, sycamores, and bigleaf maples twist toward the sky in fantastic form. Winter waves break large and powerful upon the coastal shore. And very few people are out enjoying it.

This is the time of the year to savor views, waterfalls, and those regions overrun with people during the rest of the year. With incredible vistas of the entire Bay Area, Angel Island is a prime destination between storms. In crowded and popular Point Reyes National Seashore, visitation is as light as it ever gets. Waterfalls are at their peak throughout the region. Impressive winter swells and warm, sunny stretches make the coast an inviting place. Watch the weather report closely—strong winter storms make for an intense camping experience suitable only for the properly equipped.

Spring (March–May)

The rains of winter pour into the wildflowers of spring, and open hillsides dance in a radiance of color. The riot of springtime progresses rapidly. By early to mid-March, wildflowers and new oak leaves have begun to appear at lower elevations. By the end of March, wildflowers start to peak at elevations below 500 feet. As April progresses, spring marches up the hills to higher elevations—by mid-April in a typical year, it has reached the 2,000-foot elevation, and by the end of the month has reached the highest crests of the Bay Area. In May, wildflowers continue to bloom, but the sun has already started to turn the lush green hillsides to a rustling brown.

Spring is a fabulous time throughout the Bay Area. It is virtually impossible to go wrong when selecting a destination. The coast is alive with sunshine, and wildflowers are abundant on open coastal bluffs. Fog is infrequent, though it does begin to arrive in step with the increasing temperatures of late spring.

The Marin Headlands and Point Reyes beckon. East of the Bay, one of the narrowest windows of all swings open. Regions that scorch intolerably in summer and fall are green, inviting, and flush with water. Watch the dazzling progression of spring as your elevation changes on the Ohlone Trail and its parklands. The backcountry of Henry W. Coe State Park has plentiful water sources, but hurry because they'll be gone by the end of May.

Summer (June–August)

A season of dramatic climatic contrast, summer is also vacation time for students and their families. From Memorial Day through Labor Day, visitation at Bay Area parks increases markedly. Securing a trail camp reservation at many destinations requires planning months in advance—especially for weekends and holidays—and crowds can dominate many an overnight experience. It is the time for shady inland spots, sheltering redwood forests, and lesser-traveled destinations. Campers should avoid the popular, well-known parks such as Big Basin Redwoods and Point Reyes and opt instead for lesser-traveled parks such as Pescadero Creek County Park, Butano State Park, or Austin Creek State Recreation Area.

Fall (September–November)

Following the mania of Labor Day weekend, schools reopen their doors and absorb the children and families who have filled parks all summer long. Weekends remain busy in September at many parks, but use begins to drop off markedly in October and securing a weekend spot in the shoulder month of November is generally not a problem. Weekdays are almost completely empty. The great weather and sudden reduction in crowds make fall a prime time for exploring nearly everywhere in the Bay Area. Conditions are dry and brown across much of the region, but the pleasant weather means all parks are open for outdoor play.

The Living Bay Area

For the sake of simplicity, the Living Bay Area is categorized in this book into five basic ecosystems that share common characteristics and flora: redwood forest, mixed-evergreen forest, oak woodland, chaparral, and coastal scrub. Bear in mind, however, that the Bay Area is a world of extraordinary ecological diversity; much greater detail can be found in the sources recommended in the list of sources (see page 201).

The ecosystems of the Bay Area are determined largely by one factor: the availability of water. Land farther inland bakes in stronger summer temperatures, reducing available moisture dramatically during the dry season. Regions closer to the coast receive more moisture from arriving storms, and the damp breath of summer fog provides for a year-round water supply. The following environments result, presented in order of decreasing moisture.

Redwood Forest

Redwood forest occurs in a narrow belt close to the coast where winter rainfall is abundant (30 to 60 inches annually) and summer fog is common. This damp and shady world is characterized by the majestic coast redwood *(Sequoia sempervirens)*, a tree world-famous for its size, longevity, and beauty. In the Bay Area, redwood forest occurs throughout the western Santa Cruz Mountains and fills many of the coastal drainages of the North Bay, extending as far inland as Napa and Sonoma valleys. While the majority of redwood forest has been logged over the past 150 years, numerous old-growth stands still remain.

Other moisture-loving plants join the redwoods: the drooping branches, rough bark, and feathery cones of Douglas-fir; the large spiny leaves of tanoak, particularly abundant in the understory of second-growth forest; the small pointed leaves and thick bushes of huckleberry, which dangle edible blue-black fruit in the fall; the velvety soft leaves of California hazel shrubs; and the large leaves and thin branches of bigleaf maple, common along streams and blushing gold in the fall.

Lush flora also carpets the ground: the large fronds of sword ferns, easily identified by the "hilt" at the base of their leaves; the huge fronds of chain ferns, the largest of all California ferns and found only in the wettest locations; the delicate five-finger fern, often found hanging off steep rock faces with more than five "fingers"; and a thick carpet of cloverlike redwood sorrel, whose light-intolerant leaves fold up when struck by direct sunlight. Mushrooms, including two of the world's deadliest: the death cap and destroying angel, explode from the forest floor during the wet months of winter. While animal life is abundant in the redwood forest, dense foliage makes sightings rare. Clambering orange-bellied newts and the ubiquitous banana slug are the most common fauna seen.

Mixed-Evergreen Forest

Mixed-evergreen forest is similar to redwood forest and shares many of the same flora, but does not receive enough moisture to sustain redwood trees. It commonly occurs along the margins of redwood forests and the two ecosystems often gradate into each other. It is found throughout the Santa Cruz Mountains, especially in the upper elevations; bordering the redwood forest drainages of the North Bay; covering Inverness Ridge on Point Reyes National Seashore; and in scattered moist pockets throughout the Bay Area, often on cooler north-facing slopes.

Douglas-fir is the dominant tree of mixed-evergreen forest, accompanied by its redwood-forest constituents of huckleberry, tanoak, and bigleaf maple. These are joined by the smooth peeling bark, twisting branches, and large oval leaves of madrone trees; the long, thin, and fragrant leaves of California bay trees, often arching gracefully across the forest; the gnarled forms of evergreen canyon and interior live oak, which commonly hybridize and grow both ragged-toothed and smooth-edged leaves on the same tree; and tall deciduous black oak trees, which bud out red leaves in the spring, drop golden leaves in the fall, and are easily identified by the spine-tipped lobes of their large leaves.

Oak Woodland

Oak woodland occurs where rainfall is low (15 to 25 inches annually) and summers are hot and dry. Fog is rare and provides little, if any, moisture. Extremely common in regions east of the Bay, oak woodland occurs only intermittently in the North Bay and rarely in the Santa Cruz Mountains. As conditions become progressively drier, the forest transitions from a continuous, shady cover to an increasingly open landscape dotted with solitary trees in large, grassy fields (also known as oak savanna).

This ecosystem overlaps closely with the range of gray pine, a thin wispy tree with a trunk that typically splits into several main stems. It features long (8 to 12 inches) gray-green needles in bundles of three and massive cones that often weigh more than three pounds. In damp locations along stream gullies, California bay and madrone are often joined by the mottled gray bole and twisting personage of California sycamore, characterized by huge leaves

and spiny seed balls; and by the broad, brilliantly green palmate leaves of California buckeye, the first tree to emerge with new leaves in spring (often as early as January). The buckeye is also the first to drop leaves in summer; large one-eyed (buckeyed) seed balls remain dangling on the branches. But it is the oaks that dominate.

Valley oak is the largest and most majestic of these beautiful trees, identified by its deeply lobed, 4- to 6-inch deciduous leaves with smooth margins. Hardy blue oak survives in conditions too hot and dry for other oaks and is increasingly common in the dry landscape farther east. Often occurring in pure stands, it is known by its barely lobed, wavy leaf margins and blue-green cast in late summer and fall. Other oaks include coast live oak, with its round, spiny, evergreen leaves curled into concave form; Oregon oak, with lobed leaves similar to valley oak but occurring only in scattered locations in the North Bay; and black oak, typically restricted to elevations above 2,000 feet. Spring wildflowers are dazzling in oak woodlands—a sweeping palette of color infuses the landscape from March through May. Wildlife is abundant as well, and the open forest makes sightings much easier. Deer, bobcats, wild pigs, wild turkeys, and hawks are often seen, along with a wide variety of other birdlife. Unfortunately, poison oak is extremely common in this environment as well—be watchful!

Chaparral

Chaparral grows in the driest of environments, adapted to survival in conditions intolerable for any tree. Low-lying and scrubby, chaparral offers little in the way of shade for overheating hikers and makes for difficult off-trail trekking. It flourishes on the dry slopes and

SUDDEN OAK DEATH

A scourge is sweeping through the oaks of the Bay Area, killing them by the thousands. Sudden oak death (SOD) threatens to devastate vast tracts of our natural heritage. Please do your part to prevent the spread of this epidemic.

SOD is caused by *Phytophthoraramorum*, a destructive fungus that kills the food-distributing tissue beneath the bark of infected trees. Infection can be identified by the presence of cankerous sores on the main trunk, which bleed a dark-brown or amber-colored sap and mark the locations where the fungus is doing its deadly work. As the disease weakens the tree, other organisms move in as well. Oak beetles burrow into the wood and leave a film of sawdust on the surface, joined by the black domes of another unrelated fungus. Withering away from the onslaught, the healthy-seeming foliage of an afflicted tree can turn from green to brown in a matter of weeks, signaling the tree's "sudden" death.

The fungus is currently killing three species in the Bay Area—coast live oak, tanoak, and black oak—and can affect up to 80 percent of the trees in any given stand. However, it has also been found on more than a dozen other species, including California bay, madrone, rhododendron, huckleberry, manzanita, and buckeye. These hosts are not killed by the fungus, but likely act as important vectors for the spread of the disease. So far, none of the white oak species (blue, valley, and Oregon oaks) is known to be infected.

SOD was first observed in 1995 in a small Marin County grove of tanoak trees. Within a few years, hundreds of surrounding trees were dead. As the dieback spread to other Bay Area counties, its cause remained a mystery despite increasing scientific

exposed ridges found east of the Bay, along the eastern flanks of the Santa Cruz Mountains, and in scattered eastern locations of the North Bay. Pockets of chaparral regularly appear within oak woodlands.

Shrubs of the chaparral adapt to the dry environment with small, water-retaining foliage. Coyote brush is one of the most common and occurs throughout the Bay Area in dry locations—look for the small irregular leaves often found at the end of long, bare stems, and their fuzzy white flowers in spring. Chamise sprouts a multitude of tiny, needlelike leaves along stiff woody stems and grows in thick stands. The smooth, blood-red wood of manzanita is unmistakable. Dozens of manzanita subspecies exist, each intricately twisted and blooming with tiny, bell-shaped flowers in winter and early spring.

Forty-three varieties of *Ceanothus* exist in California, many of which are found in the Bay Area. One common variety, buckbrush, grows two small waxy leaves opposite each other that are lined with a prominent mid-vein. The shrub explodes with a coating of white flowers in the spring. Other scrutiny. Only in 2000 was the *Phytophthora* fungus identified as the causal agent, a hitherto unknown species in a genus harboring the same fungus responsible for the Irish potato blight of the mid-19th century. Today, SOD has been found in nearly every county of the Bay Area and continues to spread.

The fungus is spread through three primary mediums—water, soil, and infected wood. Of these, soil is of greatest concern for Bay Area hikers, campers, and mountain bikers. Soil from afflicted areas will often contain fungal spores capable of infecting new areas. Contaminated dirt stuck to hiking boots, animals, car tires, or bicycles is easily transferred to another area on a later adventure and can spread the blight to previously unaffected areas.

To prevent the spread of SOD, please adhere to the following recommendations:

- Wash soil or mud from shoes, mountain bikes, and animals' feet prior to leaving an infected site. If this is not possible, wash them in an area at home that will not result in mud being washed directly toward other trees or waterways.

- If possible, avoid driving or parking vehicles in areas where they may accumulate contaminated soil or mud. Vehicles that have mud in the tires from an infected area should be run through a car wash.

- Do not remove plant material of any kind from an infested area.

- Avoid transporting oak wood for use in campfires as the fungus can remain active in infected dead wood for a considerable length of time.

- For more information and current updates on SOD, visit the California Oak Mortality Task Force web site at **www.suddenoakdeath.org.**

common varieties include deerbrush and blue blossom, both of which are adorned in springtime with long sprays of fragrant white, pale blue, or pink flowers. Rabbits and other small rodents hide in the thick brush, avoiding the watchful eyes of red-tailed hawks and other raptors overhead.

Coastal Scrub

Coastal scrub flourishes along the coastal margin of the Bay Area, where the ravages of salt-laden air and strong winds make life impossible for red-

woods and other interior trees. Instead, a tangled and intricate world of shrubbery exists, a wide range of species interlocking in a tight web of life.

Many plants common to chaparral environments, including coyote brush and ceanothus, thrive here as well. Joining the tangled web are the thorny vine tangles of blackberry; the abundant but inedible berries of coffee berry, which progress from green to red to black as they ripen; the vines of honeysuckle, whose terminal leaves sprout as one diamond-shape before splitting into two as it grows; the tough, spiny leaves of the diminutive scrub oak; and the hardiest of all ferns, the bracken fern, whose fronds curl under at the margins. Poison oak is extremely common in coastal scrub as well.

The treeless expanse of coastal scrub extends as far as a mile inland before the first trees appear. These include the coast live oak, cypress, and the Monterey pine, whose gnarled architecture is festooned with lopsided, smooth-scaled cones. Rabbits, deer, and bobcats are common, as is a wide variety of birdlife that finds shelter in the impenetrable brush.

Who Runs the Parks of the Bay Area?

There are more than 200 parks and preserves in the Bay Area managed by no fewer than a dozen different governing agencies. Of these, five agencies maintain facilities for overnight backpacking adventures and are consequently featured in this book. They run the gamut from federal to state to county government groups, each of which has unique procedures and regulations.

Since communication between the governing agencies is minimal, figuring out who runs what from where by what rules can be a mind-bending process. Here, each of the five featured agencies are discussed in greater detail to help you select the perfect outdoor destination.

National Park Service

The National Park Service (NPS) is a federal agency (a division of the Department of the Interior) and manages the Golden Gate National Recreation Area (GGNRA) and Point Reyes National Seashore through its Pacific West Regional Office. Dedicated to protecting the natural and historic beauty of its parklands, the NPS is generally well staffed and its facilities nicely maintained. Several excellent visitor centers are open daily for research and education.

The GGNRA includes the Marin Headlands and is the largest urban national park in the nation, protecting more than 75,000 acres of open space. Point Reyes National Seashore includes 30,000-acre Phillip Burton Wilderness, where the land is managed to maintain its wilderness qualities. Backpacking reservations are handled through the respective park visitor centers—Bear Valley Visitor Center (Point Reyes) and the Marin Headlands Visitor Center.

California State Parks

California State Parks are run by the state from its headquarters in Sacramento. In the Bay Area, state parks are scattered broadly and account for half of the trips featured in this book. Each park unit is largely a self-contained entity; they all strive to preserve parklands in as natural a condition as possible. Staffing and facilities vary widely by location, however, and the park system is in constant need of additional funding. Budgets cuts in recent years have resulted in higher fees at state parks, and caused several parks to close entirely during the off-season (roughly November through April). Expect the situation to remain in flux in the years ahead—always check in advance before embarking on a trip, especially in the off-season.

East Bay Regional Park District

The East Bay Regional Park District (EBRPD) includes both Alameda and Contra Costa counties and protects nearly 100,000 acres of open space in more than 60 designated parks. Established in 1934, it is one of the oldest regional park districts in the country and manages its lands for a range of activities, from wilderness hiking to golf courses to motorboating. It is the dog-friendliest park agency in the Bay Area, and canines can run off-leash through the undeveloped areas of almost all EBRPD lands (the Ohlone Trail is an exception). All trail camp reservations are made through the park's reservation office at 888-EBPARKS (327-2757).

San Mateo County Parks

San Mateo County Parks protect 14,000 acres in 17 parks, the smallest amount of land among the featured park districts. While the majority of its small park units are located on the northern San Francisco peninsula, a large complex of three parks in the redwood forest of the Santa Cruz Mountains—Memorial, Pescadero Creek, and Sam McDonald—provide overnight outdoor opportunities and backpacking trailheads. Pescadero Creek County Park is one of the least traveled parks in the Bay Area.

Midpeninsula Regional Open Space District

Midpeninsula Regional Open Space District is an independent special district established in 1972 for the sole purpose of preserving open space land in its natural condition. Centered along the long spine of Skyline Ridge in the Santa Cruz Mountains, the district currently includes nearly 50,000 acres of land in more than 25 preserves. Only one overnight opportunity is available—Black Mountain Trail Camp in Monte Bello Open Space Preserve.

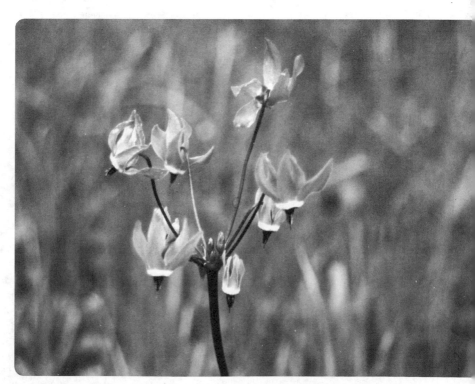

Shooting stars

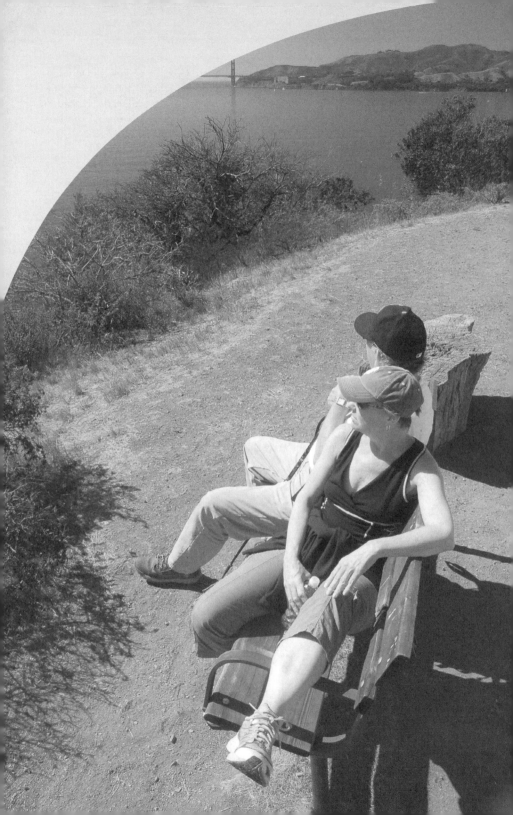

North Bay

Rolling open headlands, spectacular coastal views, and remote beaches provide a nearly irresistible allure for backpackers drawn to the power of the sea. Add in swathes of lush forest, soaring beachside cliffs of twisted geology, and more than 100 miles of easy-walking trails, and it's apparent why this region's parklands are some of the most traveled in the Bay Area.

The North Bay includes the region found north of the Golden Gate and is characterized by rugged topography and a wild coastline. A series of high ridges and peaks geographically isolates the western coastal areas from the population centers found closer to the Bay. Farther east, linear Sonoma and Napa valleys lie between mountainous ridges of volcanic rock. The region is remarkable for its large amount of easily accessible protected open space available for exploration—44 percent of Marin County is composed of parks, preserves, and other public land.

Almost all of the backpacking opportunities, however, are found in the western regions closer to the coast, with Point Reyes National Seashore and the Marin Headlands the principal destinations. Angel Island, a remarkable state park in the middle of San Francisco Bay rich in both history and astonishing views, is the one exception.

Exceptional Golden Gate and Bay views can be found all over Angel Island.

25

1 Angel Island State Park

RATINGS	Scenery **9** Difficulty **1** Solitude **1**
ROUND-TRIP DISTANCE	2.6 to 3.0 miles
ELEVATION GAIN/LOSS	+300'/–300' to Ridge Sites; +500'/–500' to East Bay and Sunrise sites
RECOMMENDED MAP	*Angel Island State Park Map* by California State Parks
BEST TIMES	Year-round
AGENCY	Angel Island State Park, Box 318, Tiburon, CA 94920, (415) 435-1915, **www.angelisland.org**. Visitor center, (415) 435-5390, is usually open 8 a.m.–sunset daily.
PERMIT	Trail camp reservations can be made for specific sites up to six months in advance (800-444-7275 or **www.reserveamerica.com**). Spring, summer, and fall weekends are usually booked far in advance. Space is generally available weekdays year-round on a first-come, first-served basis (check with the visitor center).

Highlights

In the middle of the Bay, less than 5 miles from downtown San Francisco, Angel Island rises like a jewel. Accessible only by ferry, the island offers a backpacking experience unlike any other, where vistas sweep 360 degrees around the Bay, gentle paths mingle with history, and unique rock outcrops tell unusual tales.

Hike Overview

Short and easy trails take different routes to four separate camping areas scattered around the island. The island is small—1.5 miles across at its widest—and each campsite serves as an excellent base camp for exploring the many natural and historic sites. All sites are accessible via bicycle and many of the island's trails are smooth, level, and perfect for relaxed cycling. Paved Perimeter Road rings the island in a level 5.0-mile loop and passes most historic locations. *Dogs are prohibited.*

Ferries travel to the island year-round but much less frequently in winter when views are at their most spectacular. On a winter weekday you may be the only visitor on the entire island! Weekend use picks up markedly in spring and fall, though weekdays remain quiet. The island is extremely popular every day in summer, however. Fog regularly streams over the island in summer as well, obscuring views and chilling the air. Bring a windbreaker and warm clothes year-round.

Trail Camps

A total of nine campsites and one group site are open year-round. Each campsite (described in greater detail below) accommodates up to eight people and is equipped with a nearby potable water faucet, picnic table, food locker, outhouse, and barbecue grill. There is also one additional site designated for disabled campers only. Sites are $30 per night except for Kayak Camp, which is $50. Campfires are not allowed, though charcoal may be used in the grills.

Ridge Sites are located on the windier, western side of the island and offer striking views of San Francisco, the Golden Gate Bridge, and much of

☻ Angel Island State Park

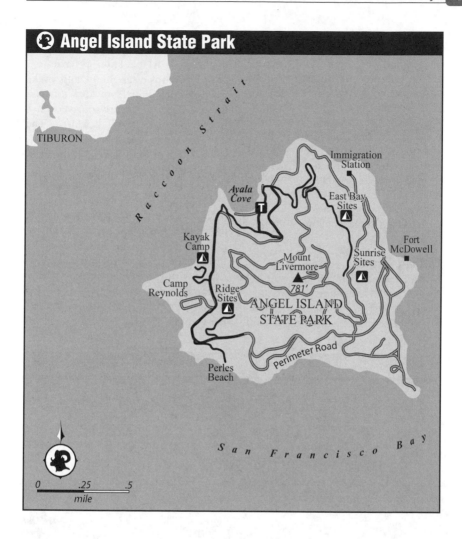

the Bay Area. Site 4 has the best views but no shelter and is totally exposed to wind. Site 5 hides beneath Monterey pine and cypress and provides good wind protection and nearby views. Site 6 is in a grassy clearing just below the ridgeline next to Battery Wallace; it has the most space and good wind protection, but no views from the site itself.

Kayak Camp is a group site (maximum 20 people) located 80 feet above a small beach on the west side of the island. The site features an open clearing (which can get soggy in winter) surrounded by coast live oaks, toyon, and coyote brush. A separate handicapped-accessible site is located just above Kayak Camp.

East Bay and Sunrise Sites are closely situated on the east side of the island and provide views of the early morning sun rising over the East Bay hills. Both camping areas are close to Mt. Livermore, Fort McDowell, and the Immigration Station, where interpretive programs are offered regularly in summer. East Bay Sites 1–3 are situated beneath the boughs of Monterey pines and coast live oaks. They provide good privacy but limited views. Site 1 is the largest, Site 2 the most secluded, and Site 3 the most open. Sunrise Sites 6–9 are packed together in a windswept, level clearing with open views to the east and no privacy among the sites; using all three together is ideal for large groups.

Getting There

A short ferry trip is required to reach Angel Island. Depending on the season, ferries depart from three locations: Tiburon, Pier 41 in San Francisco, and

Oakland and Alameda. From Tiburon, the closest and most frequently served dock, Angel Island-Tiburon ferries depart weekends year-round and make multiple trips daily from April through October; less frequently on weekdays from November through March. The terminal is on Main Street in downtown Tiburon (415-435-2131 or **www. angelislandferry.com**).

Pier 41 and Alameda and Oakland are served by Blue & Gold Fleet ferries (415-705-8200 or **www.blueandgold fleet.com**). From Pier 41 (adjacent to popular Pier 39 on San Francisco's Embarcadero), ferries depart daily year-round with increased service on weekends and during the summer. Pier 41 is the only weekday option from December through February.

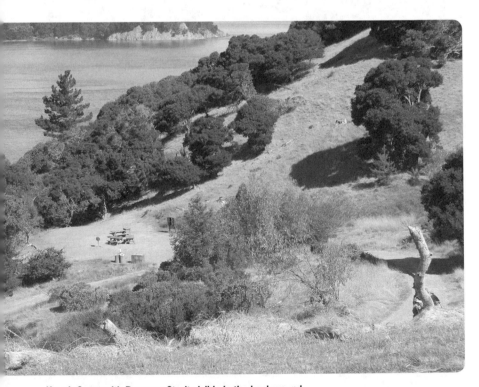

Kayak Camp with Raccoon Strait visible in the background

From Oakland and Alameda, ferries run weekends only from May through September. Terminals are located in Oakland at the foot of Clay Street in Jack London Square, and in Alameda at Gateway Center, 2991 Main Street. Service is also available once daily on weekends from May through September.

Hiking It

RIDGE AND KAYAK SITES From the ferry landing at Ayala Cove (0.0/0'), proceed to the right toward the large grassy picnic area and visitor center to register with park staff. Large Monterey pines shade the visitor center, which is housed in an original structure dating from the cove's use as a quarantine station during the early to mid-1900s (for more about the island's history, see page 30).

At the three-way junction behind the visitor center, bear right toward Camp Reynolds. Passing a few residences for state park staff and families who live on the island, the paved road soon becomes dirt and narrows as it climbs steeply via large steps to reach wide and level Perimeter Road (0.3/160'). Bear right. Epic views north to Mt. Tamalpais (2,571') and the Tiburon peninsula slowly widen to encompass San Francisco and the Golden Gate. Coast live oak, lupine, sage, coyote bush, and monkeyflower dominate the nearby dry hillsides, while pockets of bay and sword ferns grow lush on shady north-facing slopes.

Layered sandstone outcrops, which have been slightly deformed by past tectonic forces, are common on this initial stretch of trail. As the trail proceeds past the first buildings of Camp Reynolds and the junction to Kayak Camp (0.7/170'), it passes into an unusual realm of rock formed deep within the earth.

As a tectonic plate is forced beneath an adjacent continent—or subducted—it descends 10 to 30 miles into the inner layer of the earth (the mantle) where temperatures are hot enough to melt all rocks. However, since the diving plate is cool and warms slowly, some of it may not melt. Instead, portions may be altered into new rock-forms by extreme pressure, and reemerge much later at the site of the now dormant subduction zone—telltale indicators of its previous existence. Keep your eye out around Camp Reynolds for blueschist, a vibrantly dark blue stone that was created in such a way. Also striking are the altered serpentine outcrops (above Ridge Sites) and pillow basalt exposures (along Perles Beach and below Kayak Camp).

Perimeter Road passes above Fort Reynolds (an obvious access road leads down to the historic structures), then curves east to reach the junction for Perles Beach—a great place to enjoy views south toward San Francisco and the Golden Gate. The junction for Ridge sites soon follows on the left (1.3/180'). The campsites are spread out along the ridge above (1.4/200' to 270'). To access Mt. Livermore (781') from camp, head directly up the ridge behind the water tank, past the fascinating serpentine outcrops, across the first road, and all the way to Sunset Trail. The best views on the island can be found on the summit.

EAST BAY AND SUNRISE SITES After registering with park staff (see description above), proceed to Perimeter Road on the paved road leading uphill from the visitor center (0.0/0'). Turn left on Perimeter Road to reach the four-way junction with Northridge

Trail (0.4/150'), located near a picnic table beneath eucalyptus trees. (This junction also may be accessed via Northridge Trail from the ferry dock, a more direct single-track option that begins at the north end of Ayala Cove and climbs steeply beneath coast live oaks and Monterey pines.) Bear right (uphill) on single-track Northridge Trail as it begins a slow climb through the dense vegetation common on the shadier north slopes of the island. Here bay, sword fern, hazel, and wood rose join the more common coast live oak, sage, and sticky monkeyflower. Intermittent views to the north are possible across narrow Raccoon Strait, named for the 1814 repair of the British man-of-war HMS *Raccoon* in Ayala Cove— and not the critters that visit Angel Island campsites nightly.

The vegetation changes as the winding trail reaches more exposed ridge; manzanita, coyote brush, ceanothus, scrub oak, and chamise grow in this drier environment. The trail then reaches another paved road (1.0/450'). Bear left on the pavement (continuing straight on Northridge Trail leads to the island's summit). The fire road contours around to the east side of the island and soon reaches the posted junction for East Bay Sites by a large metal-roofed dome structure (1.3/400'). To reach Sunrise Sites, continue past the fenced-off water supply area and follow the road down to join yet another road (1.5/360'). Go right toward Mt. Livermore to immediately reach Sunrise Sites on the left.

Giving Back

The **Angel Island Association** supports the preservation and interpretation of history, structures, and natural resources of Angel Island State Park. Contact the association or learn more at Box 866, Tiburon, CA 94920, (415) 435-3972, or **www.angelisland.org**.

ANGEL ISLAND HISTORY

Angel Island has witnessed its share of human activity during the past 300 years. Prior to Spanish colonization it was a fishing and hunting outpost for the native Ohlone tribe. The first European to explore the island was Lt. Juan Manuel de Ayala in 1775. It became a Spanish cattle ranch during the 1840s and later housed a Union fort during the Civil War. It was an infantry camp through the late 1800s (Camp Reynolds) and in the early 1900s contained numerous gun batteries (Wallace, Ledyard, and Drew) built to protect the Golden Gate.

Through the 1940s Angel Island was a quarantine station (Ayala Cove) and processing center (Fort McDowell) for overseas troops and ships. It also held a prison site for German POWs during World War I and World War II and was an immigration station for more than 150,000 arriving Chinese, detained here from two weeks to six months while their applications for citizenship were verified. Finally in 1954 the beginnings of a state park formed at Ayala Cove and grew to encompass nearly the entire island in 1962 after the U.S. Army shut down an active NIKE missile base.

2 The Marin Headlands:
GERBODE VALLEY LOOP

RATINGS	Scenery **8** Difficulty **3** Solitude **3**
ROUND-TRIP DISTANCE	7.3 miles
ELEVATION GAIN/LOSS	+1,500'/–1,500'
RECOMMENDED MAP	*Golden Gate Hiking & Biking Waterproof Trail Map* by Map Adventures
BEST TIMES	Year-round
AGENCY	Marin Headlands, Golden Gate National Recreation Area, (415) 331-1540, **www.nps.gov/goga/mahe**
PERMIT	A free trail camp permit can be reserved up to 90 days in advance by calling the Marin Headlands Visitor Center at (415) 331-1540, which is open daily 9:30 a.m.–4:30 p.m. Summer weekends fill well in advance; permits are available most other times. Register at the visitor center by 4:30 p.m. or the permit will be cancelled; notify the visitor center ahead of time to arrange an after-hours pick-up.

Highlights

It is as it was. Rolling hills cleft by valleys, split by ridges, battered by the sea. A land of sweeping vistas, vibrant life, and dramatic geology in a protected natural world isolated from the bustle of the Bay Area. The Marin Headlands await.

Hike Overview

Hawk Camp, one of the most remote destinations in the Headlands, is accessed on a view-rich loop around untrammeled Gerbode Valley. The wide, well-graded trails circle a delightfully self-contained natural world and are a great introduction for young backpackers to the world of Bay Area backpacking opportunity. Wildflowers bloom profusely in spring; wildlife is abundant year-round.

Given the Headlands' proximity to San Francisco, crowds and bikers are common on weekends. Expect cool, breezy conditions with lots of fog during the summer months, though the oc-casional warm, sunny day does occur. Dogs are *not* permitted. It is possible to bikepack to the site via Bobcat Trail, but the full loop can't be completed on two wheels; a 1.5-mile section of Miwok Trail is closed to bikers.

Trail Camp

Hawk Camp is situated beneath a small stand of Monterey pine at an elevation of 800 feet and offers three small sites in the uppermost reaches of Gerbode Valley. Located at the end of a half-mile spur trail, it is pleasantly secluded and escapes the foot and bike traffic common throughout the Headlands. Each site accommodates a maximum of four people. An outhouse and picnic tables are available, but water is *not* provided—pack in all the water you will need. There are no reliable sources on the hike, including at the trailhead, though you can fill up at the visitor center prior to your start. Campers are limited to no more than three nights at Hawk Camp per year.

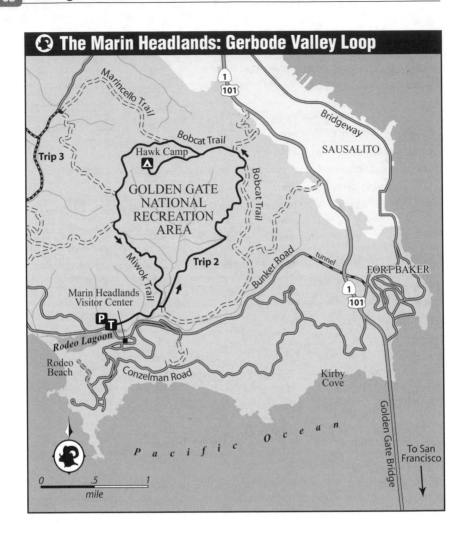

The Marin Headlands: Gerbode Valley Loop

Marincello Trail

1 101

Bridgeway

Bobcat Trail

SAUSALITO

Trip 3

Hawk Camp

Bobcat Trail

GOLDEN GATE
NATIONAL
RECREATION
AREA

Miwok Trail

Trip 2

Bunker Road

tunnel

FORT BAKER

1 101

Marin Headlands
Visitor Center

P T

Rodeo Lagoon

Rodeo
Beach

Conzelman Road

Kirby
Cove

Pacific   Ocean

Golden Gate Bridge

To San
Francisco

0   .5   1
mile

Getting There

Backpackers must first register at the visitor center. Approaching from the south, take Highway 101 to the Alexander Avenue exit (the first off-ramp north of the Golden Gate Bridge) and follow signs toward the Marin Headlands, turning left to pass through a one-lane tunnel and then continuing straight on Bunker Road for approximately 2 miles to the visitor center. Approaching from the north, take the last Sausalito exit

immediately before the Golden Gate Bridge, turn left at the stop sign, bear right up steep Conzelman Road and continue straight on this spectacular road for 3 miles to the intersection by Battery Alexander. Turn right and continue 0.5 mile to the visitor center.

After registering, bear left out of the parking lot and then immediately left again toward Fort Cronkhite to reach the trailhead on the right in a quarter mile.

Hiking It

The journey begins (0.0/20') on broad Miwok Trail, passing through open grassland punctuated with coyote brush, blackberry brambles, and a brilliant seasonal display of lupine, poppies, paintbrush, checkerbloom, irises, and other common wildflowers. Throughout the hike, watch for quail and jackrabbits in the brush, black-tailed deer and the elusive bobcat in open clearings, and red-tailed hawks and other raptors overhead. The trail briefly enters a small riparian alley and encounters a small feeder trail on the right from nearby Bunker Road (0.4/20'). Filled with willows, stinging nettle, wild cucumber vines, horsetail, elderberry, dogwood, bracken fern, vetch, and other moisture-loving plants, this dense world contrasts markedly with the surrounding dry slopes.

Continue straight on Miwok Trail to quickly reach the junction with Bobcat Trail (your return trail) on the right (0.5/30'). Remain on Miwok Trail as it turns toward the valley slopes and begins a steady climb. Passing some folded and layered chert outcrops, Miwok Trail next reaches a junction with Wolf Ridge Trail on the left (1.6/600') where views north into adjacent Tennessee Valley appear. As the trail briefly undulates along the ridgeline, look south to spot downtown San Francisco peeking over the hills. To the north, the long spine of Mt. Tamalpais slowly starts to rise above the nearby hills. Miwok Trail narrows to single-track

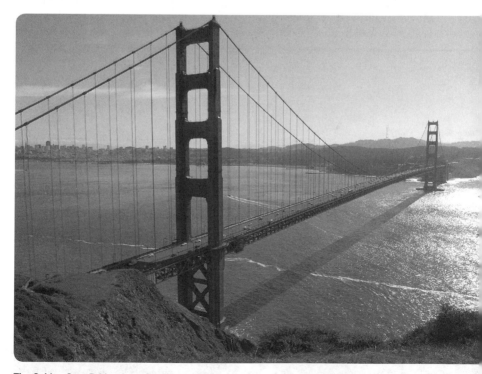

The Golden Gate Bridge from Conzelman Road

shortly before reaching the junction with Old Springs Trail.

Continue on Miwok Trail as it climbs steeply toward the FAA facilities atop Hill 1041 and stratospheric views across the Bay Area. To the south: Gerbode Valley, the Golden Gate Bridge towers, downtown San Francisco, antenna-lined San Bruno Mountain, and distant Montara Mountain (1,831'). To the east: Mt. Diablo (3,849'), the Bay Bridge, Oakland, Berkeley, and the entire East Bay hills. To the north: Mt. Tamalpais (2,578') dominates above Mill Valley, the Tiburon peninsula, and Angel Island. To the west: the vast Pacific Ocean, dimpled with the Farallon Islands on clear days.

The trail splits and rejoins around the fenced-off FAA facilities, continuing past the hilltop on Bobcat Trail as Miwok Trail splits left to descend into Tennessee Valley (2.5/1,000'). Drop-

ping from the hilltop, you next reach the junction with Marincello Trail (2.8/900')—bear right to remain on Bobcat Trail, noting the small coast live oaks below the junction. After a brief downhill, you reach the junction for Hawk Camp (3.1/780'). Bear right to head toward the small copse of trees that marks the camp location (3.7/800'). While Monterey pines are most common around camp, introduced incense cedar, eucalyptus, and a palm tree mix it up. Views stretch down San Francisco's Pacific shore to Pedro Point in southern Pacifica (a distance of nearly 20 miles).

From camp, return to the earlier junction with Bobcat Trail (4.3/780') and marvel at the completely protected world of Gerbode Valley. Now imagine that instead of this beautiful undeveloped valley before you, there were 30,000 people living in a self-contained

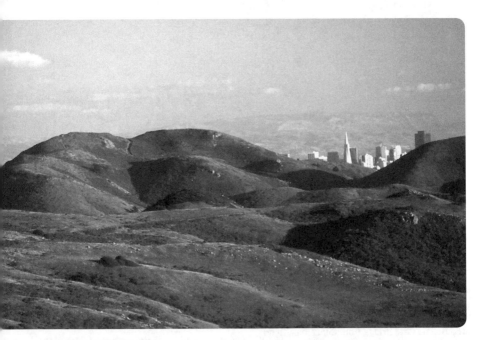

So close, yet so far away

community called Marincello. Hundreds of homes line Wolf Ridge, 19 high-rise buildings tower 16 stories tall above the valley, and schools, churches, shopping centers, and light industry complete the development.

During the 1960s, it almost happened. A master development plan was drawn up for the privately held valley, an access road (Marincello Trail) was built, and construction loomed nigh. Financial and bureaucratic delays slowed the project, however, and a key court decision in the late 1960s ultimately stopped the project altogether. The Nature Conservancy purchased the land for $6.5 million and bequeathed it to the National Park Service, which protects it for public enjoyment.

To return, follow Bobcat Trail as it dips beneath power lines and passes junctions on the left for Alta Trail (4.8/730') and Rodeo Valley Cut-off Trail (4.9/720'). As you begin the slow, descending traverse back to the trailhead, note the different vegetation that grows in the moist, protected, north-facing gullies by the trail—bay, hazel, coast live oak, elderberry, and the odd Douglas-fir can all be spotted. Bobcat Trail passes the junction with Rodeo Valley Trail (6.7/50') shortly before reaching the earlier junction with Miwok Trail (6.8/30') and the final return stretch to the trailhead (7.3/20').

Giving Back
Golden Gate National Parks Conservancy is a nonprofit membership organization dedicated to the preservation and public enjoyment of the Golden Gate National Parks. Contact the conservancy or learn more at (415) 561-3000 or **www.parksconservancy.org**.

3 The Marin Headlands:
TENNESSEE VALLEY

RATINGS	Scenery **8** Difficulty **1** Solitude **2**
ROUND-TRIP DISTANCE	1.5 miles
ELEVATION GAIN/LOSS	+250'/–250'
RECOMMENDED MAP	*Golden Gate Hiking & Biking Waterproof Trail Map* by Map Adventures
BEST TIMES	Year-round
AGENCY	Golden Gate National Recreation Area, Marin Headlands Visitor Center, (415) 331-1540, **www.nps.gov/goga/mahe**
PERMIT	A free trail camp permit can be reserved up to 90 days in advance by calling the Marin Headlands Visitor Center at (415) 331-1540, which is open daily 9:30 a.m.–4:30 p.m. Summer weekends fill well in advance; permits are available most other times. Register at the visitor center by 4:30 p.m. or the permit will be cancelled; notify the visitor center ahead of time to arrange an after-hours pick-up.

The Marin Headlands: Tennessee Valley

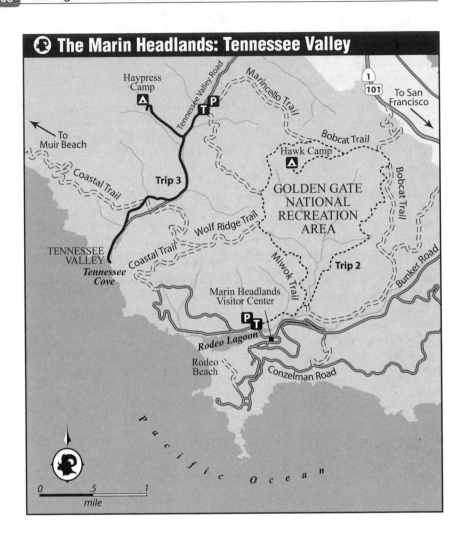

Haypress Camp

Tennessee Valley Road

Marincello Trail

To San Francisco

To Muir Beach

Bobcat Trail

Hawk Camp

Coastal Trail

Trip 3

GOLDEN GATE NATIONAL RECREATION AREA

Bobcat Trail

Wolf Ridge Trail

TENNESSEE VALLEY

Tennessee Cove

Coastal Trail

Miwok Trail

Trip 2

Bunker Road

Marin Headlands Visitor Center

Rodeo Lagoon

Rodeo Beach

Conzelman Road

Pacific Ocean

0   .5   1
mile

Highlights

Less than a mile from the trailhead, at the end of a lightly traveled spur trail, in a world secluded from everything, Haypress Camp is as close and easy as it gets. Add 3 miles of dayhiking to explore Tennessee Valley and its isolated beach at the base of 400-foot-high cliffs, and you have an outstanding adventure ideal for families and young first-time backpackers.

Hike Overview

The hike is short and easy, can be traveled by bike, and makes for an excellent year-round destination. It also offers especially good (and dramatic) geologic exposures. The main trail down Tennessee Valley is extremely popular, but Haypress Camp is a half mile removed from it and much quieter. Cool, foggy conditions are common in summer, but Haypress Camp's sheltered location protects it from much of the area's regular winds. Winter brings beautiful sunny stretches between rainstorms and a dramatic, turbulent ocean. *Dogs are prohibited.*

Trail Camp

Haypress Camp is at trail's end in the back of a small valley at an elevation of 250 feet. Eucalyptus trees provide shade and shelter from the wind for five grassy sites enclosed by a rustic zigzagging wooden fence. Adjacent to each other in a pleasant clearing, each site offers a picnic table, food locker, and two designated tent sites (maximum four people per site). Privacy is minimal. From November to March, groups can reserve all five sites at once. From April to October, no more than three sites may be reserved per group. An outhouse is available, but water is *not* provided and there are no reliable sources on the hike or at the trailhead.

Pack in all the water you will need. Campers may stay up to three nights per year.

Getting There

Backpackers must first register at the visitor center. Approaching from the south, take Highway 101 to the Alexander Avenue exit (the first off-ramp north of the Golden Gate Bridge) and follow signs toward the Marin Headlands, turning left to pass through a one-lane tunnel and then continuing straight on Bunker Road for approximately 2 miles to the visitor center. Approaching from the north, take the last Sausalito exit immediately before the Golden Gate Bridge, turn left at the stop sign, bear right up steep Conzelman Road and continue straight on this spectacular road for 3 miles to the intersection by Battery Alexander. Turn right and continue 0.5 mile to the visitor center.

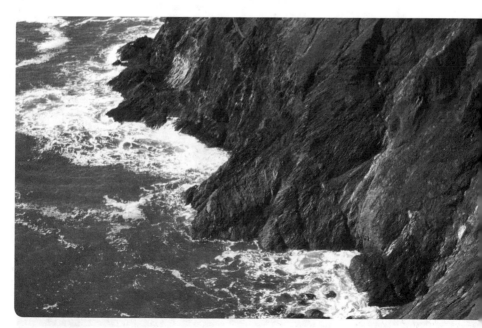

Cliffs north of Tennessee Valley

From the visitor center, return to Highway 101, head three miles north, take the Highway 1 North/Stinson Beach exit, turn left on Highway 1, and then quickly left again on posted Tennessee Valley Road. The often-crowded trailhead lot is 2 miles farther at road's end.

Hiking It

From the trailhead (0.0/200'), head down the broad path to instantly leave the developed Bay Area behind. During the early 20th century, Tennessee Valley was the domain of Portuguese dairy ranches, and the Headlands were a remote and rugged outpost divided from San Francisco by the unbridged Golden Gate (electricity did not arrive here until the 1930s). The few remaining structures in Tennessee Valley are relics of this period.

Briefly paralleling a moist, willow-choked riparian alley, the trail quickly reaches the posted junction for Hay-press Camp (0.3/140'). Bear right toward camp and continue to the back of the valley to find the sites (0.7/250'). Bulbous rock outcrops and a lone Douglas-fir protrude from the coastal scrub of surrounding slopes. Use trails wend everywhere for exploration. An ephemeral camp-side trickle provides habitat for large sword and chain ferns, coffee berry, and poison oak. For being less than a mile from the trailhead, the sense of isolation is remarkable.

To visit the beach, return to the main trail and turn right. Heading downvalley, you pass a private residence on the left and continue past junctions for the Coastal Trail to reach the small pocket beach at trail's end; a single-track, hikers-only alternate trail

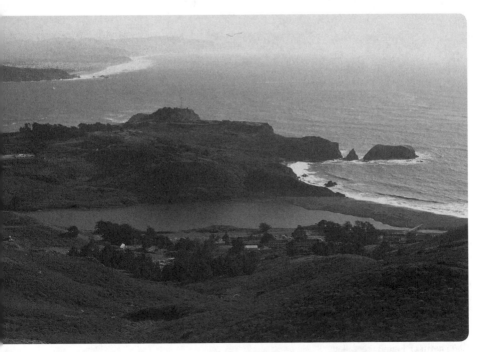

Rodeo Lagoon and Beach are visible from locations throughout the Headlands.

splits and rejoins the main trail along the way. As you proceed, marvel at the 1,000-foot-high ridges to the north and south that together hem in this remarkable coastal valley.

Tennessee Valley is named for the 1853 shipwreck of the SS *Tennessee,* which foundered here on its way to San Francisco from Panama. The ship sank, but all of its nearly 600 passengers and 14 chests of gold made it to safety. The vessel's huge cast-iron engine can occasionally be seen at the south end of the beach during low tides.

North of the cove, a peephole pierces towering cliffs of layered red chert and clearly discernible pillow basalts

(learn more about Bay Area geology on page 13). Use trails clamber up the steep slopes, where stomach-queasing vertical drops and an abandoned bunker await discovery. To the south, a fascinating realm of multihued boulders can be accessed at lower tides. Return the way you came.

Giving Back
Golden Gate National Parks Conservancy is a nonprofit membership organization dedicated to the preservation and public enjoyment of the Golden Gate National Parks. Contact the conservancy or learn more at (415) 561-3000 or **www.parksconservancy.org**.

4 Point Reyes:
WILDCAT CAMP AND ALAMERE FALLS

RATINGS	Scenery **7** Difficulty **4** Solitude **3**
ROUND-TRIP DISTANCE	11.0 miles
ELEVATION GAIN/LOSS	+2,000'/–2,000'
RECOMMENDED MAP	*Point Reyes National Seashore Trail Map* by Tom Harrison Maps
BEST TIMES	Year-round
AGENCY	Point Reyes National Seashore, Bear Valley Visitor Center, (415) 464-5100, **www.nps.gov/pore**
PERMIT	Trail camp reservations are required. Call (415) 663-8054. See "Trail Camp" (page 40) for more information.

Highlights
This hike winds along the coastal edge of Point Reyes National Seashore, passing lakes, epic viewpoints, and a short side trip to Alamere Falls, which tumbles 40 feet directly onto Wildcat Beach. The beach is arguably the most remote stretch of accessible coastline in the Bay Area, flanked by cliffs of

twisted geology and easily accessed in only one spot—Wildcat Camp.

Hike Overview
The trip begins at the Palomarin Trailhead near the southern end of Point Reyes and travels north along broad, easy-walking Coast Trail. Ocean views are common and expansive as the route winds along coastal bluffs, passes

ⓦ Point Reyes: Wildcat Camp and Alamere Falls

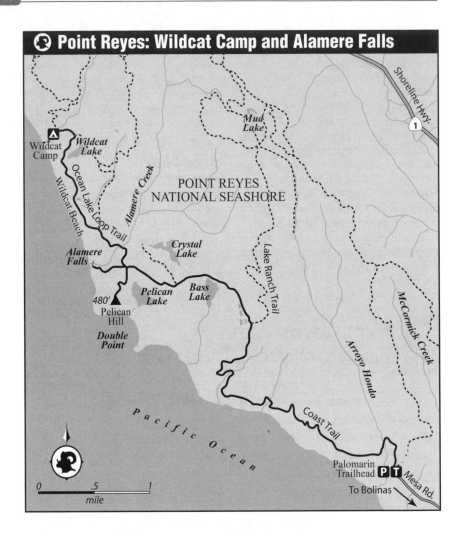

several freshwater lakes, and ends at Wildcat Camp—the most remote camping area in Point Reyes. Summer means fog, crowds, and unseasonably cold conditions, but long hours of daylight. Spring explodes with wildflowers, lush green hillsides, and highly variable weather. Fall provides frequent sunshine, warm days, and a golden, dry landscape. Winter offers crystalline air and powerful surf, but is interspersed with torrential storms.

Trail Camp

Perched on a bluff above 2 miles of pristine beach, adjacent to a singular point of coastal access, and ensconced in the heart of nature's domain, Wildcat Camp is a delight. And yet its attributes are also the very things that make Wildcat Camp the least accessible of the backcountry camps: Fog is frequent, coastal winds are constant, and strong winter storms rip into the unprotected camp. Bring a sturdy tent year-round and know how to pitch it tautly; guylines can be essential in the windiest conditions.

Wildcat Camp offers seven sites, including four group sites. The sites are well-spaced and often hidden behind tall grass or brush, providing a sense of privacy and solitude. Sites 1–4 are the group sites (capacity 15–25, depending on the site). All four are large, open, and essentially identical; the only difference is their proximity to the water and bathroom—Sites 1 and 2 are closer. Sites 5–7 are smaller (capacity six), but are located closer to cliff's edge and offer majestic coastal views; they are somewhat protected by patches of coyote brush—Site 5 is the most sheltered.

Pit toilets, picnic tables, food lockers, and a faucet of nonpotable water are provided; bring a filter or other water-treatment method. Marauding skunks, raccoons, and foxes nightly scavenge the campground and have been known to invade tents with food (and sleeping people) inside—secure all food and scented items inside the provided food lockers. *Wood fires are prohibited,* although charcoal may be used in the provided grills. Campstoves are permitted. Driftwood fires are allowed on the beach below high tide line; a special permit from Bear Valley Visitor Center is required.

Camping is by permit only (violators are subject to a $150 fine). Reservations may be made up to three months in advance (to the day) by calling (415) 663-8054, 9 a.m.–2 p.m. Monday through Friday. Reservations can also be made in person at the Bear Valley Visitor Center during open hours or by fax (download the appropriate form at **www.nps.gov/pore**). If sites are available, walk-in registration is possible for same-day departures.

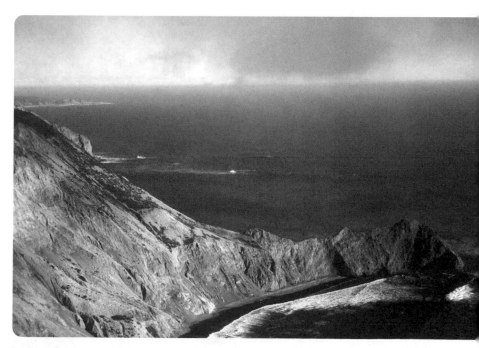

Double Point

Campsites cost $15 per night for 1–6 people, $30 per night for 7–14 people, and $40 per night for 15–25 people. Permits must be obtained from the Bear Valley Visitor Center prior to leaving on your trip. It is open 9 a.m.–5 p.m. weekdays, and 8 a.m.–5 p.m. weekends and holidays. After-hours pick-up is allowed—permits are placed in a wooden box by the information board in front of the visitor center.

Planning is crucial to secure a site at Wildcat Camp. From April through October, it is difficult to obtain a campsite for a weekend night less than two months in advance. During summer months, every day is usually booked several weeks ahead of time.

Getting There

You'll need to first visit the Bear Valley Visitor Center to pick up your permit. To get there, head to the small town of Olema on Highway 1. From the intersection of Highway 1 and Sir Francis Drake Boulevard in downtown Olema, proceed north on Highway 1 and make an immediate left on Bear Valley Road. In 0.5 mile, turn left again to reach the visitor center.

To reach the trailhead, return to Highway 1, head south 9 miles to the Olema-Bolinas Road junction (immediately prior to the northern edge of Bolinas Lagoon), and turn right. The turnoff is usually not posted—keep an eye out for it. In 1.2 miles, the road reaches a T-junction—go left, continuing on Olema-Bolinas Road for 0.5 mile before turning right again on Mesa Road. Follow Mesa Road 4.6 miles to the large parking lot at road's end, passing a Coast Guard radar station and the Point Reyes Bird Observatory along the way. The last 1.3 miles are unpaved.

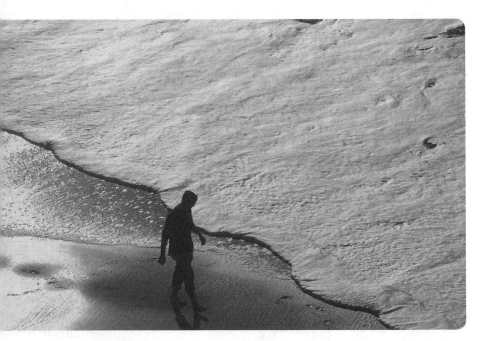

Coastal contemplation

THE WEATHER OF POINT REYES

Point Reyes National Seashore experiences a range of climatic conditions unlike anywhere else in the Bay Area. From April through October, thick blankets of fog bury low-lying coastal regions. Strong onshore winds are common. The encroaching fog encounters a formidable obstacle at Inverness Ridge, however, and is often unable to overcome the thousand-foot rise in elevation. As a result, eastern regions bask in more frequent sunshine. On a typical summer day, conditions at the Bear Valley Visitor Center may be sunny, calm, and 80 degrees, while just a few miles west it will be foggy, breezy, and in the 50s.

In the winter, conditions change. Incoming storms are forced over Inverness Ridge, dropping increased moisture at higher elevations. As a result, ridgelines are the wettest places in the region, with the upper slopes of Inverness Ridge averaging twice the precipitation of the coast and Olema Valley. Average daily temperatures, however, fluctuate little year-round. Warm, sunny days occur every month of the year, but you should always prepare for the most common conditions: wind, wet, and temperatures in the 50s.

Hiking It

From the trailhead (0.0/280'), the wide path immediately enters a thick eucalyptus grove where wild cucumber vines twine and a few enormous trees hulk in ethereal whispers—one huge Hydralike specimen is by far the largest eucalyptus visited in this book. Good views south open up as the trail next winds along open blufftops; the Farallon Islands are visible southwest on a clear day.

The trail turns inland, crossing two small creek gullies choked with willows, horsetail, watercress, monkeyflowers, and bracken ferns before resuming ocean views. At the third significant creek gully, the trail heads farther inland, climbing over a small divide to the Lake Ranch Trail junction (2.2/570'). Continuing ahead on Coast Trail, you meander through a dense forest of young Douglas-fir as the trail passes several swampy ponds

full of lily pads before reaching views of larger Bass Lake ahead. Gradually descending along its northern shore, the trail leads to a short spur path on the left and an open area that provides excellent opportunities for a break and swim. (Be aware that Bass Lake is popular with nudists.)

Beyond Bass Lake, the trail soon passes a junction for unexciting Crystal Lake (3.0/500') before traversing above beautiful Pelican Lake. Point Reyes and the long curving arc of beach and coastal bluffs appear north. Descending, you reach a spur junction on your left (3.6/290') immediately after views north become obscured by the coastal bluffs. This small trail climbs 0.3 mile to the top of Pelican Hill (480') and the north end of Double Point, a spectacular and recommended side trip. Far-reaching views sweep south and north from the summit, while the inaccessible cove beach below is often filled with hundreds of hauled-out seals.

The rock of this area is Monterey shale, a sequence of sedimentary layers up to 8,000 feet thick that were deposited on the granite bedrock of Point Reyes National Seashore over the past 20 million years. In the region around Double Point, this shale has become involved in a huge landslide nearly four miles long and at least a mile wide. As this huge block of land slips slowly toward the sea, depressions are formed that fill with freshwater lakes such as Pelican and Bass lakes.

Immediately past the junction for Pelican Hill, another unposted spur trail splits left (3.7/270'). This overgrown and brushy path leads 0.3 mile down to Alamere Falls, unseen until the very end, where some scrambling is required to reach the stream and its series of cascades. Some additional—and more challenging—scrambling is required to reach the beach via a rocky chute. The bluffs are impressive, and the tilted, exposed layers of Monterey shale are spectacular south of the falls.

From the falls, you can hike 1.3 miles north along the sands of Wildcat Beach to reach Wildcat Camp, a unique beach backpacking experience and a more direct and level route to camp. Note, however, that sections of the beach may be impassable during high tides and heavy surf—and there is no exit from the beach between Alamere Falls and Wildcat Camp. The narrow

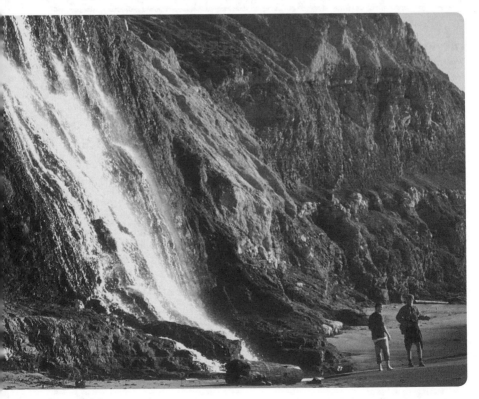

Alamere Falls

beach section immediately north of the falls is a good indication. If waves are reaching the cliff base, do *not* proceed.

To reach Wildcat Camp via the inland route, return to Coast Trail and head north into the drainage of Alamere Creek where alder, elderberry, and thimbleberry thrive in the moister environment. Contouring past the creek, Coast Trail next reaches the junction with Ocean Lake Loop (4.2/240'). While both trails lead equidistantly to camp, bear left on more scenic Ocean Lake Loop Trail (perhaps returning on Coast Trail for variety).

Single-track Ocean Lake Loop Trail drops gently to bank around marshy Ocean Lake before climbing abruptly to reach a bench with great views of Wildcat Beach. After descending past brush-lined and inaccessible Wildcat Lake, you reach Coast Trail rejoining from the right (5.3/220'). Continue left on Coast Trail. The open field of Wildcat Camp appears before a final drop through a thick corridor of willow and vetch deposits you at camp (5.5/70').

Giving Back

The nonprofit **Point Reyes National Seashore Association** works to preserve the extraordinary wilderness of Point Reyes and to educate the public about the environment. Contact the association or learn more at (415) 663-1200 or **www.ptreyes.org**.

---

5 Point Reyes:
SKY CAMP TO PALOMARIN

RATINGS	Scenery **7** Difficulty **4** Solitude **3**
ONE-WAY DISTANCE	15.4 miles
ELEVATION GAIN/LOSS	+2,300'/–2,980'
RECOMMENDED MAP	*Point Reyes National Seashore* by Tom Harrison Maps
BEST TIMES	Year-round
AGENCY	Point Reyes National Seashore, Bear Valley Visitor Center, (415) 464-5100, **www.nps.gov/pore**
PERMIT	Trail camp reservations are required. Call (415) 663-8054. See "Trail Camps" (page 47) for more information.

Highlights

This hike travels the length of Point Reyes' Phillip Burton Wilderness, from lush mixed-evergreen forests atop thousand-foot ridgelines to dramatic ocean views along the coastline. A point-to-point journey, this adventure takes in many of the park's best highlights, including secluded beaches, far-reaching views, and eye-popping cliff-side geology. And it cruises mostly downhill for the first half of the journey. The only drawback is the long car shuttle required to leave vehicles at either end of the hike.

🌀 Point Reyes: Sky Camp to Palomarin

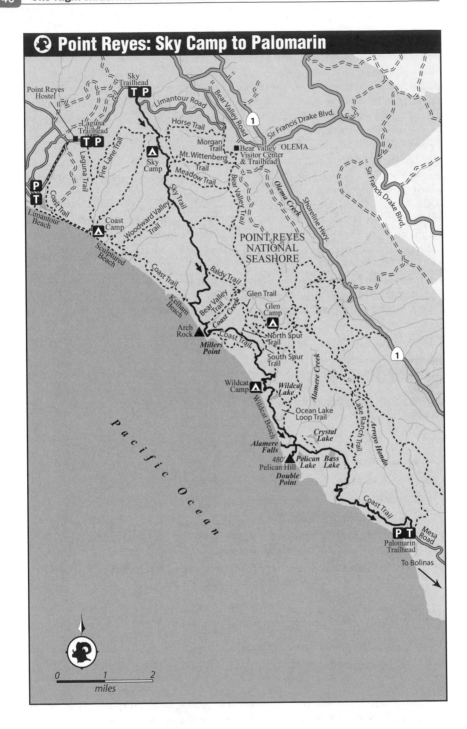

Point Reyes Hostel

Sky Trailhead
T P

Limantour Road

Laguna Trailhead
T P

Horse Trail

Bear Valley Road

Sir Francis Drake Blvd.

①

Morgan Trail

Mt. Wittenberg

■ Bear Valley Visitor Center & Trailhead   OLEMA

Fire Lane Trail

Sky Camp

Meadow Trail

Laguna Trail

P T

Coast Trail

Limantour Beach

Coast Camp

Woodward Valley Trail

Sky Trail

Sir Francis Drake Blvd.

Olema Creek

Shoreline Hwy.

Bear Valley Trail

POINT REYES NATIONAL SEASHORE

Sculptured Beach

Coast Trail

Baldy Trail

Bear Valley Trail

Coast Creek

Glen Trail

Glen Camp

Kelham Beach

Arch Rock ▲

Coast Trail

Millers Point

North Spur Trail

South Spur Trail

①

Wildcat Camp

Wildcat Lake

Alamere Creek

Lake Ranch Trail

Wildcat Beach

Ocean Lake Loop Trail

Crystal Lake

Arroyo Hondo

Alamere Falls

480' Pelican Hill

Pelican Lake   Bass Lake

Double Point

Coast Trail

P T   Mesa Road

Palomarin Trailhead

To Bolinas

Pacific Ocean

0   1   2
miles

Hike Overview

The trip begins at Sky Trailhead at the northern edge of the wilderness, reaching Sky Camp in a short and easy 1.3 miles. The route next descends a forested ridgeline to the coastline, meeting Coast Trail near the midpoint of the wilderness area. From there, you travel along the coastal margin toward Wildcat Camp and secluded Wildcat Beach, completing your coastside journey at Palomarin Trailhead near the southern edge of the wilderness.

Trail Camps

Two trail camps are available on this hike: Sky Camp and Wildcat Camp. The recommended overnight spot is Wildcat Camp, located near the journey's midway point. Sky Camp is only 1.3 miles from the starting trailhead— an excellent option for a late start on a two-day, two-night adventure.

A thousand feet high with views to match, **Sky Camp** features pleasantly secluded sites tucked amid coastal scrub and Douglas-firs. Only 3 miles from the Pacific shore, the camp resounds with the echo of breaking waves and the closer-in vocalizations of scampering California quail. Sky Camp has 12 sites, including one large group site. Expansive views are available from many points in the area, but vistas from the sites themselves are limited by surrounding brush. Site 2, the group site (capacity 25), offers less privacy but good views and easier access to water and bathrooms. Sites with higher numbers are farther from the water and toilet facilities but offer more seclusion.

Perched on a bluff above 2 miles of pristine beach, adjacent to a singular point of coastal access, and ensconced in the heart of nature's domain, **Wildcat Camp** is a delight. And yet its attributes are also the very things that make Wildcat Camp the least accessible of the backcountry camps: Fog is frequent, coastal winds are constant, and strong winter storms rip into the unprotected camp. Bring a sturdy tent year-round.

Wildcat Camp offers seven sites, including four group sites. The sites are well-spaced and often hidden behind tall grass or brush, providing a sense of

---

PLANTS AND FORESTS OF POINT REYES

Weather shapes the dramatic ecology of Point Reyes National Seashore. The high ridges harbor dense mixed-evergreen forest nourished by heavy winter rains and dense summer fog. A rich tapestry of ferns and elderberry and huckleberry bushes fill an open understory beneath majestic Douglas-fir. California bay, hazel, and coast live oak thicken the forest on the lower slopes.

Along the coast, regular winds and salty air preclude forest growth, giving rise instead to thick, low-lying coastal scrub predominated by coyote brush, coffee berry, and blackberry vines. Wildflowers begin to appear in late February and become increasingly abundant over the ensuing spring months; Douglas iris, California poppy, bush lupine, checkerbloom, and tidy tips are particularly abundant.

Be watchful throughout Point Reyes for the toxic leaves of poison oak and wicked needles of stinging nettle—both are common nemeses throughout the backcountry.

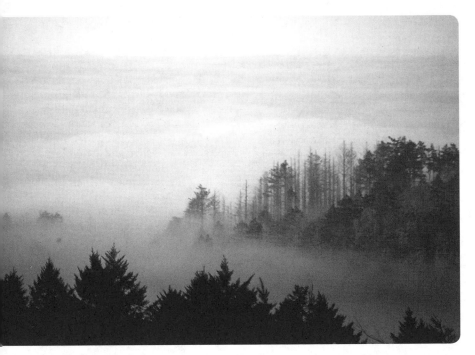

A sea of fog below Sky Camp

privacy and solitude. Sites 1–4 are the group sites (capacity 15–25, depending on the site). All four are large, open, and essentially identical; the only difference is their proximity to the water and bathroom—Sites 1 and 2 are closer. Sites 5–7 are smaller (capacity six), but are located closer to the cliff's edge and offer majestic coastal views; they are somewhat protected by patches of coyote brush—Site 5 is the most sheltered.

Pit toilets, picnic tables, food lockers, and water faucets are provided at both trail camps (potable at Sky, nonpotable at Wildcat; bring a filter or other water-treatment method). Marauding skunks, raccoons, and foxes nightly scavenge the campground and have been known to invade tents with food (and sleeping people) inside—secure all food and scented items inside the provided food lockers. *Wood fires are prohibited,* though charcoal may be used in the provided grills. Campstoves are permitted. Driftwood fires are allowed on the beach below high tide line, if you get a special permit from Bear Valley Visitor Center.

Camping is by permit only (violators are subject to a $150 fine). Reservations may be made up to three months in advance (to the day) by calling (415) 663-8054, 9 a.m.–2 p.m. Monday through Friday. Reservations can also be made in person at the Bear Valley Visitor Center during open hours or by fax (download the appropriate form at **www.nps.gov/pore**). If sites are available, walk-in registration is possible for same-day departures.

Campsites cost $15 per night for 1–6 people, $30 per night for 7–14 people, and $40 per night for 15–25 people. Permits must be obtained from the Bear Valley Visitor Center prior to leaving on your trip. It is open 9 a.m.–5 p.m. weekdays, and 8 a.m.–5 p.m. weekends and holidays. After-hours pick-up is allowed—permits are placed in a wooden box by the information board in front of the visitor center.

Planning is crucial to secure a site, especially at Wildcat Camp. From April through October, it is difficult to obtain a site at Wildcat Camp for a weekend night less than two months in advance. During summer months, every day is usually booked several weeks ahead of time. Sky Camp is also popular, though space may be available on shorter notice.

Getting There

You'll need to first visit the Bear Valley Visitor Center to pick up your permit. To get there, head to the small town of Olema on Highway 1. From the intersection of Highway 1 and Sir Francis Drake Boulevard in downtown Olema, proceed north on Highway 1 and make an immediate left on Bear Valley Road. In 0.5 mile, turn left again to reach the visitor center.

To reach the starting trailhead, take Bear Valley Road 1.5 miles north of the visitor center to Limantour Road, turn left, and follow it west for 3 miles to the Sky Trailhead parking lot, located on the left.

To reach the ending trailhead from the visitor center, return to Highway 1 and head south 9 miles to the Olema-Bolinas Road junction (immediately prior to the northern edge of Bolinas Lagoon) and turn right. The turnoff is usually *not* posted—keep an eye out for it. In 1.2 miles, the road reaches a T-junction—go left, continuing on Olema-Bolinas Road for 0.5 mile

before turning right again on Mesa Road. Follow Mesa Road 4.6 miles to the large parking lot at road's end. The last 1.3 miles are unpaved.

Hiking It

Before you begin, note the bishop pines to the left of the gate at Sky Trailhead (0.0/670'). Distinguished by their clusters of two needles, bishop pines are a rare species, found only along a narrow coastal strip within a few miles of the ocean. They favor the well-drained soils weathered from the granite rock of the northern Point Reyes peninsula. The trail crosses the geologic divide between this granitic soil and the soil weathered from the Monterey shale that underlies most of the wilderness, and is one of the best places in Phillip Burton Wilderness to see these unique trees.

The broad trail quickly ascends beneath drooping Douglas-fir branches. Coyote brush, blackberry, elderberry, thimbleberry, hazel, bracken fern, sword fern, and stinging nettle constitute impenetrable thickets along the edges of the trail. Coast live oaks appear intermittently as well, their trunks bearded by green mosses. As the trail continues to climb, note the burn marks on the trunks of some trees. Soon blackened snags protrude from bare slopes to the right, and the fire zone is revealed.

Sky Trail formed a critical defense line during the 1995 Vision Fire, providing a staging area and access for fire-fighting trucks and equipment. While flames charred the trees west of Sky Trail, the forest east of the trail was largely saved. Bishop pines are serotinous—they need the heat from wildfires to open their tightly sealed cones and release the seeds of future generations. Fire also clears out the brushy understory that might otherwise impede the growth of young trees, and provides a generative ashy, nutrient-rich soil. Without regular wildfires, bishop pines would not survive as a species—most mature trees seldom live longer than 100 to 150 years before succumbing to old age and disease. The proliferation of young bishop pines to the west of the trail demonstrates this natural ecologic succession.

As you continue past the burn zone, the trail enters an increasingly moist mixed-evergreen forest and reaches a junction with Fire Lane Trail on the right (0.7/1,060') and then Horse Trail on the left (0.8/1,040'). Immediately past Horse Trail on the left is an outcrop of layered Monterey shale (topped by huckleberry bushes), illustrative of the rock type that underlies most of the wilderness area. Remain on Sky Trail as it descends slightly, briefly parallels the burn line again, and then reaches Sky Camp (1.3/1,020').

From Sky Camp, head south on broad Sky Trail to reach the junction with Mt. Wittenberg and Meadow trails (1.9/1,120'). Bear right on Sky Trail to immediately pass beyond the Vision Fire zone and enter a wonderful stretch of mature mixed-evergreen forest. Douglas-firs tower overhead and strain moisture from fog flowing over Inverness Ridge, keeping the environment moist and green through the rain-free summer months. Water condenses on the trees' foliage, falls to the ground, and provides liquid sustenance for a vibrant understory (as much as a third of total year-round moisture here comes from fog drip). Mossy branches and tree-bound ferns droop above abundant elderberry, huckleberry, blackberry tangles, and sword ferns. Poison oak and stinging nettle appear sporadically. In September huckleberry

bushes explode with small and delicious blue-black berries.

You pass the junction for Woodward Valley Trail (2.6/890') as you continue straight on Sky Trail, climbing briefly to next reach the junction with Old Pine Trail (2.9/1,020'). Stay on Sky Trail as it gently descends through a final stretch of green forest before cresting a small rise; here, the landscape transitions to coastal scrub as you approach the junction with Baldy Trail (4.3/870'). Remain on Sky Trail as it descends toward the increasingly visible ocean. After first passing along the margin of the Vision Fire where burnt snags still protrude, the trail reaches a small saddle where coyote brush covers the thick low-lying coastal scrub landscape.

Continue your steady descent past coast live oaks, bay trees, stinging nettle, and a final sampling of mixed-evergreen forest. At last the trail makes its steepest drop on two switchbacks to the junction with Coast Trail (5.8/130'). Turn left and follow wide and sandy Coast Trail south toward Arch Rock. Shortly before you reach Bear Valley Trail (6.3/110'), a use path splits right toward scenic Arch Rock.

Follow the short spur trail to the cliff's edge atop Arch Rock itself. A wonderful picnic stop on calm days, the open blufftop provides views that stretch north along adjacent Kelham Beach to Point Resistance and beyond. On the south side of Arch Rock, a well-worn, narrow, and precarious use trail switchbacks tightly down into the mini-gorge of Coast Creek to reach sea level and fabulous views of the Arch itself. At low tide, you can access Kelham Beach through the Arch. South, a small pocket beach stretches a short distance to Millers Point and makes for fun exploring as well.

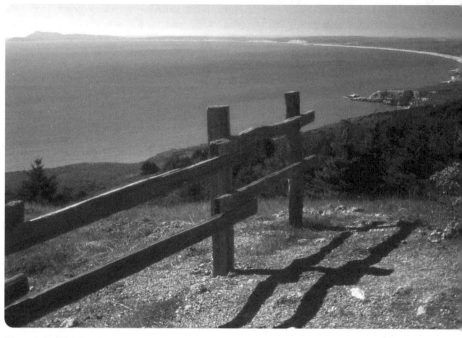

The sweep of Drakes Bay

To continue to Wildcat Camp, return to Coast Trail and head south. The route crosses Coast Creek among alders and elderberry, then curves briefly around the slopes before climbing to the open ridgeline above. Increasingly expansive views open up as the trail reaches 300 feet in elevation and encounters a use path on the right. A short 20-yard detour leads to a small knoll and gravestone marker for Clem Miller. As a local congressman, Miller was a great advocate for the creation of the national seashore and worked tirelessly to achieve the reality. Millers Point below is named in his honor.

Return to Coast Trail and continue your ascent along the ridgeline. Views become ever more thrilling as you climb. The trail finally levels out at 750 feet at one of the farthest-reaching viewpoints in the entire wilderness. Wildcat Beach and its southern terminus at Double Point are visible south. Looking north, the long curving arc of Limantour Beach and Drakes Beach terminates in the prominent mass of Point Reyes itself (9 miles away). Just out of sight, Coast Camp and the northern wilderness boundary are located where the bluffs end at the south end of Limantour Beach. Just beyond nearby Arch Rock, Kelham Beach stretches north to Point Resistance. (The bald slopes past Point Resistance were denuded by the 1995 Vision Fire.) On clear days, the sharp points of the Farallon Islands are visible to the southwest. When the weather provides exceptional visibility, you can spot the three lumpy rocks of the seldom-seen North Farallones to the west-southwest.

The single-track route levels out and reaches the junction with North Spur Trail (7.7/740'). Remain on Coast Trail as it abandons the beautiful vistas and enters a dense coastal scrub world of coyote brush, coffee berry, and blackberry and honeysuckle vines. The trail parallels the headwaters of a deep creek drainage, then gently ascends to the junction with South Spur Trail (8.3/840'). Bear right on Coast Trail as it turns south.

Once again you enjoy ocean views before turning east above the deep valley holding Wildcat Camp at its mouth. Wildcat Lake and Pelican Hill are visible down the coast to the south. Shrubs and dense fields of poison oak line the trail as it curves down and past a knobby octopus of a Douglas-fir to the junction with broad Stewart Trail (9.2/420'). Turn right and follow the wide fire road of Coast Trail as it

winds through a thick creek forest of bay and Douglas-firs. Leaving canyon bottom, you switchback steeply down past huge coffee berry bushes and willows to arrive at the open blufftop of Wildcat Camp (9.9/40').

From here, it is possible to hike 1.3 miles south along the sands of Wildcat Beach to reach Alamere Falls, a unique beach backpacking experience and a more direct and level route to your next destination. Note, however, that sections of the beach can be impassable during high tides and heavy surf, and that there is *no* exit between Wildcat Camp and Alamere Falls. Also be aware that the scramble up the bluffs by Alamere Falls is mildly precarious and not for the faint of heart. To continue inland instead, follow the Coast Trail as it climbs through a thick corridor of willow and vetch to reach the Ocean Lake Loop Trail (10.1/220').

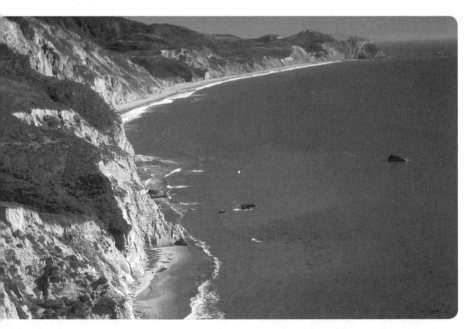

Wildcat Beach

WILDLIFE OF POINT REYES

A variety of native and introduced species live on Point Reyes. A dozen native marine mammals, 37 land mammals, and 45 percent of all bird species in North America have been sighted here. Native black-tailed deer are populous, regularly seen, and easily identified by their namesake appendage. Two introduced deer species also live here: axis deer, native to India and identified by its reddish-brown coat interspersed with white spots; and fallow deer, native to Europe and easily distinguished by its large mooselike antlers and white color. Small mammals roam and scurry throughout; campers are guaranteed a nightly visit from scavenging skunks, raccoons, and gray foxes.

Along the coast, hauled-out harbor seals are common on many beaches—the inaccessible cove at Double Point usually has a sizeable community. California gray whales migrate south past Point Reyes on their way to Baja each winter and north to the Gulf of Alaska in spring. The southern migration peaks in mid-January, the northern in mid-March. Watch for their spouts from coastal viewpoints throughout the wilderness. Remember that it is illegal to disturb marine mammals onshore. If they are altering their behavior because of your presence, you are too close.

Bear right on the Ocean Lake Loop Trail, a more scenic alternative that rejoins the Coast Trail in 1.1 miles. The narrower path ascends past brush-lined and inaccessible Wildcat Lake, reaches a bench with views north to Wildcat Beach, and then drops to bank around marshy Ocean Lake. A gentle rise returns you to the Coast Trail (11.2/240'). Bear right on the Coast Trail and descend into the Alamere Creek drainage, where alder, elderberry, and thimbleberry thrive in a moister environment.

The route curves around the stream valley, begins climbing, and reaches an unposted spur trail on the right (11.7/270'). This overgrown and brushy path leads 0.3 mile down to Alamere Falls, unseen until the very end; scrambling is required to reach the stream and its series of cascades, which end as a sheet of water tumbling directly onto the beach below. The rocky chute that leads down to the ocean requires some difficult scrambling. The bluffs are impressive, and the tilted exposed layers of Monterey shale are spectacular south of the falls.

Return to the Coast Trail and continue south, immediately reaching another unposted spur trail on the right (11.8/290'). The small trail climbs 0.3 mile to the top of Pelican Hill (480') and the north end of Double Point, another recommended side trip. Far-reaching views look south and north from the summit. An inaccessible cove beach below is often filled with hundreds of hauled-out seals.

The rock of this area is Monterey shale, a sequence of sedimentary layers up to 8,000 feet thick that were deposited on the granite bedrock of Point Reyes National Seashore over the past 20 million years. In the region around

Double Point, this shale has become involved in a huge landslide nearly four miles long and at least a mile wide. As this huge block of land slips slowly toward the sea, depressions form and fill with freshwater lakes such as Pelican and Bass lakes.

From here, the Coast Trail makes a rising traverse above beautiful Pelican Lake and passes a junction for unexciting Crystal Lake on the left (12.4/500'). Next up is larger Bass Lake, which provides the hike's best freshwater swimming opportunity; a short spur path leads to an open area on its north shore. (Be aware that Bass Lake is popular with nudists.) Continuing, Coast Trail gradually rises above the lake and then winds through a dense forest of Douglas-fir punctuated by several swampy ponds. You pass Lake Ranch Trail on

the left (13.2/570'), drop over a small divide, and curve around a creek gully choked with willows, horsetail, watercress, and bracken ferns. Several more small creeks follow as the trail winds near the open blufftops. Good views south open up as you proceed. Just before reaching the trailhead (15.4/280'), the trail enters a thick eucalyptus grove where a few enormous trees hulk; one huge Hydralike specimen watches your final steps home.

Giving Back
The nonprofit **Point Reyes National Seashore Association** works to preserve the extraordinary wilderness of Point Reyes and to educate the public about the environment. Contact the association or learn more at (415) 663-1200 or **www.ptreyes.org**.

6 Point Reyes:
COAST CAMP TO GLEN CAMP LOOP

RATINGS	Scenery **6** Difficulty **5** Solitude **3**
ROUND-TRIP DISTANCE	16.9 miles
ELEVATION GAIN/LOSS	+2,500'/–2,500'
RECOMMENDED MAP	*Point Reyes National Seashore* by Tom Harrison Maps
BEST TIMES	Year-round
AGENCY	Point Reyes National Seashore, Bear Valley Visitor Center, (415) 464-5100, **www.nps.gov/pore**
PERMIT	Trail camp reservations are required. Call (415) 663-8054. See "Trail Camps" (page 55) for more information.

Highlights
From remote beaches to wave-washed promontories, lush forests to panoramic ridgelines, this hike has it all.

Hike Overview
The journey begins along the sands of Limantour Beach, meandering along the coastal margin to reach nearby

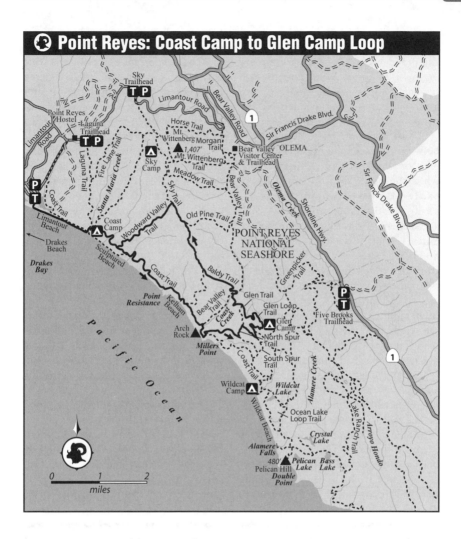

Point Reyes: Coast Camp to Glen Camp Loop

Coast Camp. From there, it travels several miles along ocean bluffs and past remote beaches to reach Arch Rock, then continues inland to reach wooded Glen Camp. On the return, you travel through lush ridgeline forest along Sky Trail before dropping back to the coast.

Trail Camps

Two trail camps are located along this hike: Coast and Glen camps. Coast Camp is easiest to access—only 1.5 miles from the trailhead—and is a mecca for large family groups and anybody looking for the shortest route to an overnight backcountry experience. Located behind a small rise at the south end of Limantour Beach, the camp marks the beginning of the striking bluffs and headlands that characterize the wilderness coastline. Sculptured Beach, a fascinating stretch of cliffs, crevices, and wave-washed promontories, is a short stroll south of camp and beckons visitors to explore its low-tidal zone. Wind and fog are regular companions at Coast Camp; a strong tent is recommended for the common northwest winds.

Coast Camp provides 14 sites split between two separate areas. Two sites are for large groups (capacity 25), while the other sites are smaller (capacity 6). Tucked within the coastal scrub, Sites 1–7 offer privacy and some are sheltered from the incessant winds (Sites 1–4 offer ocean views). Higher numbered sites are located farther from the water and restrooms; site 7 offers the greatest seclusion. Sites 8–14 are spread around a large clearing, offer minimal privacy or shelter from the winds, and are much closer to the water and restroom. Sites 10 and 14 are farther back in the valley and offer some shelter, while Sites 8–9 and 11–13 are entirely exposed, close to the main trail, and in high-traffic areas. Sites 8 and 13 are the group sites.

At the hike's midpoint, **Glen Camp** is the most sheltered of Point Reyes' four backcountry camps, tucked within forest and free from the incessant winds that whistle over much of the seashore.

It is a good place to camp during times of inclement weather and makes an ideal base camp for exploring the wide variety of nearby trails. Glen Camp lacks views and its tightly spaced sites can feel crowded on busy weekends, but space is often available here when other trail camps are full.

Glen Camp offers 12 small sites around an open clearing (there are no group sites). Sites vary greatly in privacy and shade. Sites 1–2 are pleasantly shaded, are located closest to the bathroom and water faucets, and offer decent privacy (though toilet aroma may assault the nose at times). Sites 3–4 are located adjacent to a monstrous coast live oak, which provides some shade and privacy. Sites 5–8 hide on the brushy slopes above the clearing; all offer decent privacy and some shade. Sites 9–12 surround the clearing with little to no shelter from the sun or fellow campers—Site 10 is totally exposed in the middle of camp.

Pit toilets, picnic tables, grills, food lockers, and potable water faucets are provided at both trail camps. Marauding skunks, raccoons, and foxes nightly scavenge the campground and have been known to invade tents with food (and sleeping people) inside—place

THE VISION FIRE

In October 1995 a major human-caused wildfire burned more than 12,000 acres of Point Reyes National Seashore, including a large segment of northern Phillip Burton Wilderness. Sparked from the smoldering embers of an illegal campfire atop Mt. Vision, the fire spread rapidly over the dry hillsides. In the wilderness area, the fire reached as far south as Sky Trail and left regions north heavily charred. Today the land is rapidly recovering. Young trees, especially bishop pines, are everywhere, though you can still expect to see burnt tree skeletons throughout the fire zone.

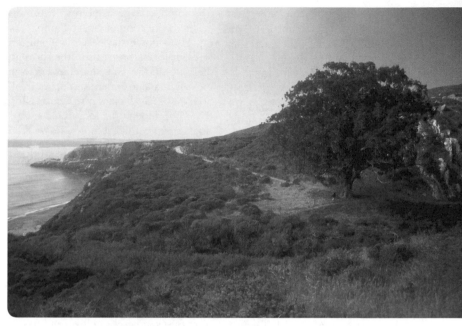

Giant eucalyptus above Kelham Beach

all food and scented items inside the provided food lockers. *Wood fires are prohibited;* charcoal may be used in the grills. Campstoves are permitted.

Camping is by permit only (violators are subject to a $150 fine). Reservations may be made up to three months in advance (to the day) by calling (415) 663-8054, 9 a.m.–2 p.m. Monday through Friday. Reservations can also be made in person at the Bear Valley Visitor Center during open hours or by fax (download the appropriate form at **www.nps.gov/pore**). If sites are available, walk-in registration is possible for same-day departures.

Campsites cost $15 per night for 1–6 people, $30 per night for 7–14 people, and $40 per night for 15–25 people. Permits must be obtained from the Bear Valley Visitor Center prior to leaving on your trip. It is open 9 a.m.–5 p.m. weekdays, and 8 a.m.–5 p.m. weekends and holidays. After-hours pick-up is allowed—permits are placed in a wooden box by the information board in front of the visitor center.

Planning is crucial. From April through October, it is difficult to obtain a campsite for a weekend night with less than two months in advance—though Glen Camp is often the last backcountry camp to fill.

Getting There

You'll first need to visit the Bear Valley Visitor Center to pick up your permit. Head to the small town of Olema on Highway 1.

From the intersection of Highway 1 and Sir Francis Drake Boulevard, proceed north on Highway 1 and make an immediate left on Bear Valley Road. In 0.5 mile, turn left again to reach the visitor center.

To reach the trailhead, take Bear Valley Road 1.5 miles north of the visitor center, turn left on Limantour Road, and follow it west for 7 miles. Immediately prior to reaching the main Limantour Beach parking lot at road's end, go left and follow the road 0.4 mile to the southernmost parking lot in the area. Parking space is limited. If the lot is full, park in the main lot and begin along the beach there.

Hiking It

Head toward the water from the trailhead (0.0/30'), following the obvious path past common members of the coastal scrub plant community: coyote brush, coffee berry, blackberry, lupine, yarrow, ceanothus, cow parsnip, and a few creekside alders. On clear days, Chimney Rock is visible to the west across Drakes Bay, marking the east end of the Point Reyes Headlands. To the south, a large eucalyptus tree indicates the location of Coast Camp.

Head down the beach, keeping an eye out for harbor seals in the surf and herons, ducks, and shorebirds in the nearby marshy wetlands. You can follow the beach all the way to Coast Camp (1.5/50'), though the loose sand makes for strenuous going at times. Coast Trail offers easier walking, and can be accessed just past the marsh where a lone bishop pine rises from the sandy dunes, about halfway to Coast Camp.

From Coast Camp (1.5/50'), continue south on broad Coast Trail as it climbs above the small valley and attains the blufftop. For the next 4 miles, Coast Trail travels atop the headlands; cliffs and steep drainages hem the coastline below. The trail curves around Santa Maria Creek, the first of several creek gullies, and passes the Woodward Valley Trail on the left (2.1/180').

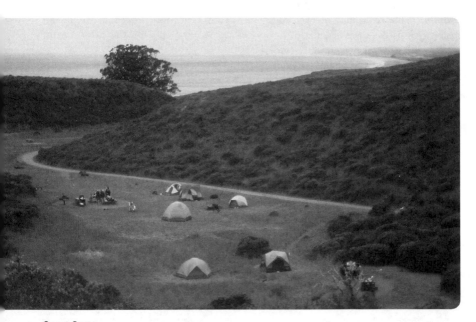

Coast Camp

The Coast Trail next encounters a wide junction (2.3/150') that provides access to a small cove at the south end of Sculptured Beach, a worthwhile side trip. Follow the narrow path and stairway down to the ocean, where outcrops of Monterey shale are dramatically overtopped by the loosely consolidated Drakes Bay Formation. At low tide, it is possible to travel from here to Coast Camp past the many formations of Sculptured Beach. Caution is in order—*there is no exit from the beach to escape encroaching waves.*

Back heading south on the Coast Trail, the route loops around a small creek and passes through an area affected by the 1995 Vision Fire, which burned more than 12,000 acres in the central wilderness area; blackened snags jut from the coastal scrub. Hardy coyote brush and bush lupine predominate in the regenerating landscape, joined intermittently by sage and morning glory. The trail curves around several more small drainages, then gradually descends to reach an enormous eucalyptus by another creek. A remnant of U Ranch, this gargantuan tree marks the access point for Kelham Beach (4.9/100'), a remote and cliff-lined strand. From the beach, views peer south toward the sea stacks offshore from nearby Arch Rock and beyond to distant Double Point.

Continuing south on the Coast Trail, you pass Sky Trail on the left (5.1/130') shortly before reaching the Bear Valley Trail near Arch Rock (5.6/110'). Take the time to visit this distinctive landmark, readily accessed by the many paths that crisscross the area. The view from its open blufftop is excellent, stretching north along adjacent Kelham Beach to Point Resistance and beyond. On the south side of Arch Rock, a well-worn but precari-

ous path descends into the mini-gorge of Coast Creek. At low tide, you can walk through the arch to access Kelham Beach to the north. To the south, a small pocket beach stretches a short distance to Millers Point.

Southbound Coast Trail next crosses Coast Creek and attains an open ridgeline. Expansive views open up as the trail climbs to 300 feet in elevation and encounters a path on the right, where a short 20-yard detour leads to a small knoll and gravestone marker for Clem Miller, a local congressman who advocated for the creation of the national seashore. Millers Point below is named in his honor. The views become more thrilling as you continue the ridgeline ascent. You eventually level out at one of the best vistas in the entire seashore.

Looking north, the long curving arc of Limantour Beach and Drakes Beach terminates in the prominent mass of Point Reyes itself. On clear days, the sharp points of the Farallon Islands are visible to the southwest. On days of exceptional visibility, you can spot the three lumpy rocks of the seldom-seen North Farallones to the west-southwest. To the south, Wildcat Beach and its southern terminus at Double Point are visible.

Just past the viewpoint, you encounter North Spur Trail (7.0/760'). Turn left, take North Spur Trail inland to Glen Trail (7.3/720'), then bear right and proceed on level Glen Trail to Glen Camp Loop Trail on the left (7.7/720'). Follow Glen Camp Loop Trail past Greenpicker Trail on the right (7.9/700') and slowly descend through a young forest. Glen Camp becomes visible below shortly before the trail banks right and drops steeply into camp (8.4/540').

From Glen Camp, your journey continues on Glen Camp Loop Trail, which narrows to single-track as it rises briefly past eucalyptus and huckleberry bushes and then traverses above a deep gully. The trail skirts a clearing, crosses a small stream, and meets Glen Trail (9.3/460'). Turn right and follow Glen Trail, which briefly runs level and offers a glimpse of the ocean, then descends through mixed-evergreen woods to emerge in a clearing of coastal scrub and coast live oak. The trail curves right, drops parallel to Coast Creek into a lush riparian world, and reaches the junction with Baldy and Bear Valley trails by a bike rack (9.9/170').

Climb out of Bear Valley on Baldy Trail, which switchbacks through lush forest before beginning a steady ridgeline ascent. Views open up into the deep drainage of Bear Valley as you continue upward to reach Sky Trail (11.1/870'). Bear right on Sky Trail, soon leaving

coastal scrub behind as you slowly rise into lush mixed-evergreen forest. Douglas-firs and huckleberry bushes predominate in the often moist environment. You pass Old Pine Trail on the right (12.5/1,020'), then descend briefly to reach Woodward Valley Trail (12.8/890').

Bear left to begin the return descent to Coast Camp on Woodward Valley Trail. Burnt and dead trees appear as the trail descends through untouched virgin forest and fire-blackened snagscapes that were created by the flames of the 1995 Vision Fire. The gradient steepens abruptly as the trail passes into a burned zone marked by spottier undergrowth and fire-blackened trunks. After switchbacking downward, the path levels and follows the contour above the fully scorched drainage of Santa Maria Creek (north). Here you have far-reaching southern views; Point Resistance, the offshore sea stacks by

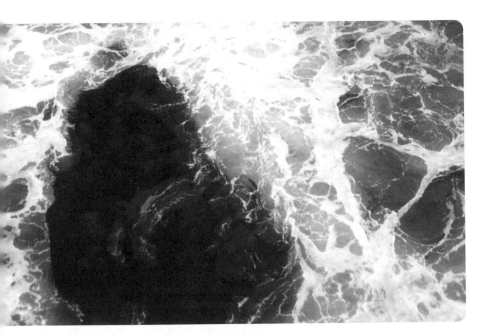

Ocean mosaic

Arch Rock, and more distant Wildcat Beach are all visible.

After entering the open world of coastal scrub, the trail descends its final switchback past numerous outcrops of Monterey shale and reaches Coast Trail (14.8/180'). Bear left (north) on Coast Trail as it winds around Santa Maria Creek and then descends into Coast Camp (15.4/50') for your beachside return to the trailhead (16.9/30').

Enjoy the sand underfoot as you savor one last stroll by the sea.

Giving Back

The nonprofit **Point Reyes National Seashore Association** works to preserve the extraordinary wilderness of Point Reyes and to educate the public about its environment. Contact the association or learn more at (415) 663-1200 or **www.ptreyes.org**.

7 Point Reyes:
BEAR VALLEY LOOP

RATINGS	Scenery **6** Difficulty **5** Solitude **3**
ROUND-TRIP DISTANCE	15.8 miles
ELEVATION GAIN/LOSS	+2,000'/–2,000'
RECOMMENDED MAP	*Point Reyes National Seashore* by Tom Harrison Maps
BEST TIMES	Year-round
AGENCY	Point Reyes National Seashore, Bear Valley Visitor Center, (415) 464-5100, **www.nps.gov/pore**
PERMIT	Trail camp reservations are required. Call (415) 663-8054. See "Trail Camps" (page below) for more information.

Highlights

Explore the full spectrum of Point Reyes National Seashore on this loop hike, which tours the lush forest atop the peninsula's highest ridgelines, descends past far-reaching views, and then explores the salt-swept coastline before returning inland via Bear Valley.

Hike Overview

The trip begins at Bear Valley Visitor Center and quickly ascends Inverness Ridge via Horse Trail, a heart-pounding start to the adventure. After visiting Sky Camp, your route descends through the emerald forest along Sky Trail to reach the coast near dramatic

Arch Rock. Some of the seashore's best coastal views follow as you ascend along the coastline before turning inland toward Glen Camp and the return route through Bear Valley. Pitch a tent at Sky Camp and Glen Camp for a relaxing two-night journey; for an overnight trip, Glen Camp is near the midpoint of the hike.

Trail Camps

Two trail camps are available on this hike: Sky Camp and Glen Camp. The recommended overnight spot is Glen Camp, located near the journey's midway point. Sky Camp is 3.4 miles from the starting trailhead and is an excellent

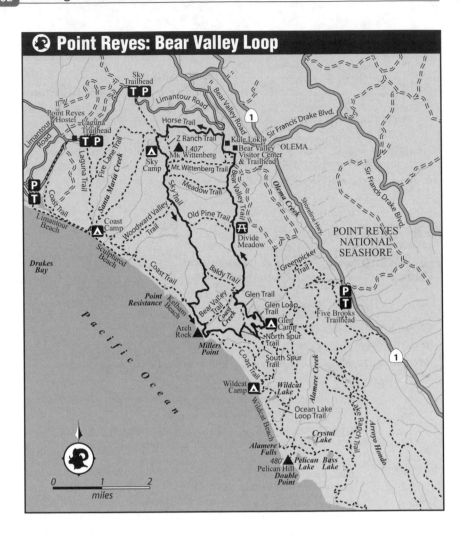

Point Reyes: Bear Valley Loop

option for a late start or a leisurely two-night adventure.

A thousand feet high with views to match, **Sky Camp** features pleasantly secluded sites tucked amid coastal scrub and Douglas-firs. Only 3 miles from the Pacific shore, the camp resounds with the echo of breaking waves and the closer-in vocalizations of scampering California quail. Sky Camp has 12 sites, including one large group site. Expansive views are available from many points in the area, but able from many points in the area, but vistas from the sites themselves are limited by surrounding brush. Site 2, the group site (capacity 25), offers less privacy but good views and access to water and bathrooms. Sites with higher numbers are located farther from the water and toilet facilities but offer more seclusion.

Tucked within forest at the hike's midpoint, **Glen Camp** is free from the incessant winds that whistle over much of the seashore and is a good place to camp during times of inclement weather. The trail camp lacks views and its tightly spaced sites can feel crowded on busy weekends, but space is often available here when other trail camps are full. Twelve small sites are situated around an open clearing (there are no group sites). They range from good to lousy and vary greatly in privacy and shade. Sites 1–2 are pleasantly shaded, are closest to the bathroom and water faucets, and offer decent privacy (though toilet aroma may assault the nose). Sites 3–4 are adjacent to a monstrous coast live oak, which provides some shade and privacy. Sites 5–8 hide on the brushy slopes above the clearing; all offer decent privacy and some shade. Sites 9–12 sit amidst the clearing with little to no shelter from the sun or fellow campers—Site 10 is totally exposed in the middle of camp.

Pit toilets, picnic tables, grills, food lockers, and potable water faucets are provided at both trail camps. Marauding skunks, raccoons, and foxes nightly scavenge the campground—secure all food and scented items in the provided food lockers. *Wood fires are prohibited;* charcoal may be used in the grills. Campstoves are permitted.

Camping is by permit only (violators are subject to a $150 fine). Reservations may be made up to three months in advance (to the day) by calling (415) 663-8054, 9 a.m.–2 p.m. Monday through Friday. Reservations can also be made in person at the Bear Valley Visitor Center during open hours or by

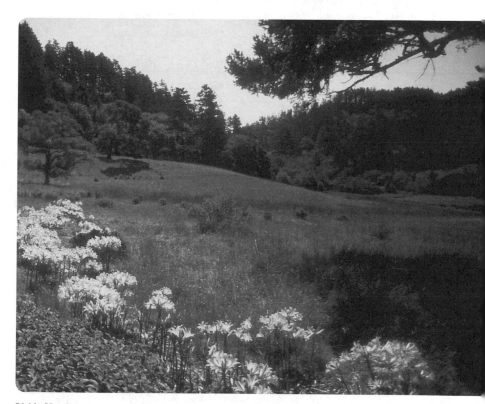

Divide Meadow

GEOLOGY OF POINT REYES

Point Reyes National Seashore is a migrant piece of land. Its deepest bedrock is granite, formed in Southern California approximately 85 million years ago. When the San Andreas Fault became active 28 million years ago, pieces of the North American continent located west of the emergent fault began to slowly migrate north at the rate of two to three centimeters per year. These landmasses traveled hundreds of miles over the ensuing millennia. One was granitic Point Reyes, which became covered by thick, waterborne sediments while submerged beneath the sea for almost 10 million years on its journey north.

Roughly 4 million years ago, a slight change in the geometry of the San Andreas Fault system increased compression on either side of the fault, pushing Point Reyes (and most of the Coast Ranges) well above sea level. Erosion then began stripping away the overlying sediment, exposing the erosion-resistant granite found on northern Inverness Ridge, Tomales Point, and Point Reyes itself. In Phillip Burton Wilderness, most of the granite is still deeply buried beneath the thick layers of sediment known as the Monterey shale. A few isolated outcrops of granite can be found on Horse Trail north of Sky Camp, but Monterey shale composes most geologic exposures (including many spectacular seaside cliffs).

In some coastal sections of the northern wilderness, however, the Drakes Bay Formation overlays Monterey shale. Deposited atop the Monterey shale in a shallow sea environment roughly 8 million years ago, it is loosely consolidated and shows no obvious layering. This formation is dramatically exposed at Sculptured Beach by Coast Camp.

---

fax (download the appropriate form at www.nps.gov/pore). If sites are available, walk-in registration is possible for same-day departures.

Campsites cost $15 per night for 1–6 people, $30 per night for 7–14 people, and $40 per night for 15–25 people. Permits must be obtained from the Bear Valley Visitor Center prior to leaving on your trip. It is open 9 a.m.–5 p.m. weekdays, and 8 a.m.–5 p.m. weekends and holidays. After-hours pick-up is allowed—permits are placed in a wooden box by the information board in front of the visitor center. Plan at least several weeks ahead of time to secure a site, longer for weekends and summer weekdays.

Getting There

The hike begins at the Bear Valley Visitor Center, where you'll pick up your overnight permit. To get there, head to the small town of Olema on Highway 1. From the intersection of Highway 1 and Sir Francis Drake Boulevard in downtown Olema, proceed north on Highway 1 and make an immediate left on Bear Valley Road. In 0.5 mile, turn left again to reach the visitor center. Park in one of the large parking lots and proceed to the obvious gate that marks Bear Valley Trail.

Public transportation is also available to the trailhead. Marin Transit (**www.marintransit.org**) offers daily service to Bear Valley Visitor Center from the San Rafael Transit Center.

Hiking It

From the Bear Valley Trailhead (0.0/80'), head north on Morgan Trail, which runs parallel to the fenced margin of Morgan Horse Farm and quickly passes Woodpecker Trail on the left (0.1/170'). Established to breed and train horses for national parks around the country, Morgan Horse Farm once had a herd of nearly 80 animals. Today individual parks maintain their own stables, and Morgan Horse Farm keeps only a few horses for trail patrol and maintenance in the seashore.

The trail soon enters a mixed-evergreen forest of Douglas-fir, tanoak, and bay, and reaches the junction for Kule Loklo (0.4/170') by a massive tanoak. (The short side trip to Kule Loklo leads to a reconstructed village of the Miwok Indians, the area's prior inhabitants.) Continue on Morgan Trail, which gently descends to Horse Trail by a wooden bridge (0.6/90'). Turn left on Horse Trail and prepare to ascend!

As you start the climb, look for the sinuous limbs of coast live oaks twining among the drooping branches of bay trees and stout trunks of Douglas-firs. Stinging nettle, fuzzy-leaved hazel bushes, blackberry tangles, soft thimbleberry leaves, and wood and sword ferns fill the understory. Wreaths of poison oak climb the trees. The single-track trail becomes steep and rutted as it steadily climbs to 900 feet, where it

briefly levels out. Granite rocks can be found here in the trail, part of Point Reyes' bedrock core.

After a final ascent, Horse Trail crests Inverness Ridge, contours south through a more open area, and passes Z Ranch Trail on the left (2.5/1,110'). Continuing on Horse Trail, you walk past some loose, layered outcrops of Monterey shale, which caps the bedrock granite throughout most of the wilderness area. Horse Trail ends at the wide fire road of Sky Trail (2.9/1,050'). Turn left on Sky Trail and cruise into Sky Camp (3.4/1,020').

Continue south past Sky Camp on easy-cruising Sky Trail, which soon passes Mount Wittenberg and Meadow trails on the left (4.0/1,120') and enters a section of mature mixed-evergreen forest. Douglas-firs tower overhead and strain moisture from the fog, keeping the environment lush and green year-round. Moss-bearded branches and tree-bound ferns droop above abundant elderberry, huckleberry, blackberry tangles, and sword ferns. In September, the huckleberry bushes dangle with abundant—and deliciously edible—blue-black berries.

Sky Trail next passes Woodward Valley Trail on the right (4.7/890') and climbs briefly to reach Old Pine Trail on the left (5.0/1,020'). Remain on Sky Trail as it gently descends and then crests a small rise where the surrounding environment transitions to low-lying coastal scrub. Here Baldy Trail splits left (6.4/870') to drop into Bear Valley, but you remain on Sky Trail and descend toward the increasingly visible ocean. The route passes a few burnt snags—remnants of the 1995 Vision Fire, which burned 12,000 acres of the seashore—and reaches a small saddle cloaked with coyote brush. The descent continues, becoming steeper near the end as it makes a final drop via two switchbacks to reach Coast Trail (7.9/130').

The continuing hike bears left (south) on wide and sandy Coast Trail, which quickly leads to Bear Valley Trail and the nearby promontory of Arch Rock (8.4/110'). (A right turn on Coast Trail leads 0.2 mile to an enormous eucalyptus situated by a small creek, the access point for Kelham Beach, a remote strand of cliffs and sandy solitude.) Take the time to visit the open blufftop of Arch Rock, readily accessed by the many paths that crisscross the area. The view is excellent, stretching north along adjacent Kelham Beach to Point Resistance and beyond. On the south side of Arch Rock, a well-worn but precarious path descends into the mini-gorge of Coast Creek. At low tide, you can walk north through the arch to access Kelham Beach. To the south, a small pocket beach stretches a short distance to Millers Point.

Heading south on Coast Trail, your continuing route crosses Coast Creek and then climbs to the open ridgeline. Expansive views open up as the trail climbs to 300 feet and encounters a path on the right, where a short 20-yard detour leads to a small knoll and gravestone marker for Clem Miller, a local congressman who advocated fiercely for the creation of the national seashore. Millers Point below is named in his honor. Coast Trail continues its ascent along the ridgeline, and the views become ever more thrilling. Your climb eventually levels out at one of the best views in the seashore.

To the north, the long curving arc of Limantour Beach and Drakes Beach terminates in the prominent mass of Point Reyes itself. On clear days, the sharp points of the Farallon Islands are visible to the southwest. When the weather provides exceptional visibility, you can spot the three lumpy rocks of the seldom-seen North Farallones to the west-southwest. Wildcat Beach and its southern terminus at Double Point are visible to the south.

Just past the viewpoint, you encounter North Spur Trail (9.8/760'). Turn left, take North Spur Trail inland to Glen Trail (10.0/720'), then bear right and proceed on level Glen Trail to Glen Camp Loop Trail on the left (10.4/720'). Follow Glen Camp Loop Trail past Greenpicker Trail on the right (10.5/700') and slowly descend through a young forest. Glen Camp becomes visible below shortly before the trail banks right and drops steeply into camp (11.2/540').

From Glen Camp, your journey continues on Glen Camp Loop Trail, which narrows to single-track as it rises briefly past eucalyptus and huckleberry bushes and then traverses above a deep gully. The trail skirts a clearing, crosses a small stream, and meets Glen Trail (12.1/460'). Turn right and follow Glen Trail, which briefly runs level and offers a glimpse of the ocean, then descends through mixed-evergreen woods to emerge in a clearing of coastal scrub and coast live oak. The trail curves right, drops parallel to Coast Creek into a lush riparian world, and reaches Bear Valley Trail by a bike rack (12.7/170').

Turn right on the broad trail and head inland alongside alder-choked Coast Creek. The arching branches of massive bay trees shade your journey to Divide Meadow (14.2/320'), a pleasant rest stop. Ringed by coast live oaks, the meadow sits on the divide between the Olema Valley and Coast Creek watersheds and is the only low-elevation gap through Inverness Ridge. A hunting lodge owned by the Pacific Union Hunting Club of San Francisco once sat in the northwest corner, a backcountry base for pursuing bears and mountain lions from the 1890s until the Great Depression. The lodge has long since been removed; two huge introduced Monterey pines and a few patches of exotic pink flowers are all that remain.

Continue on Bear Valley Trail and enter one of the seashore's most majestic forests. California bay, alders, and tanoak thrive. Mighty Douglas-firs, each unique in form and character, rise above. Bracken ferns, thimbleberry, blackberry tangles, sword ferns, elder-berry, five-finger ferns, and gooseberry grow abundantly beneath their crooked branches. On your way out, you pass Meadow Trail (15.0/150') and Mount Wittenberg Trail (15.6/80') on the left, then emerge into a more open landscape. Bear Valley Trailhead is just ahead (15.8/80').

Giving Back

The **Point Reyes National Seashore Association** works to preserve the extraordinary wilderness of Point Reyes and to educate the public about the environment. Contact the association or learn more at (415) 663-1200 or **www.ptreyes.org**.

8 Point Reyes:
TOMALES BAY BOAT-IN CAMPING

RATINGS	Scenery **8** Difficulty **5** Solitude **8**
ROUND-TRIP DISTANCE	4 to 12 miles
ELEVATION GAIN/LOSS	Negligible
RECOMMENDED MAP	*Point Reyes Hiking & Biking Waterproof Trail Map* by Map Adventures
BEST TIMES	Spring through fall
AGENCY	Point Reyes National Seashore, Bear Valley Visitor Center, (415) 464-5100, **www.nps.gov/pore**
PERMIT	Camping permit is required. Call (415) 663-8054. See "Trail Camps" (page 69) for more information.

Highlights

Remarkable wildlife and scenery highlight the Bay Area's only backcountry boat-in camping destination: Tomales Bay. Sandwiched between Point Reyes and the mainland, this remarkable body of water shelters more than a dozen beaches along its western margin where intrepid paddlers can camp along remote and sandy shores.

Trip Overview

First, you'll need a sea kayak or other appropriate, nonmotorized boat. You can provide your own or rent one from a local outfitter; Blue Waters Kayaking (415-669-2600, **www.bwkayak.com**) has locations in both Inverness and Marshall.

Tomales Bay is sheltered from ocean waves and suitable for most paddlers.

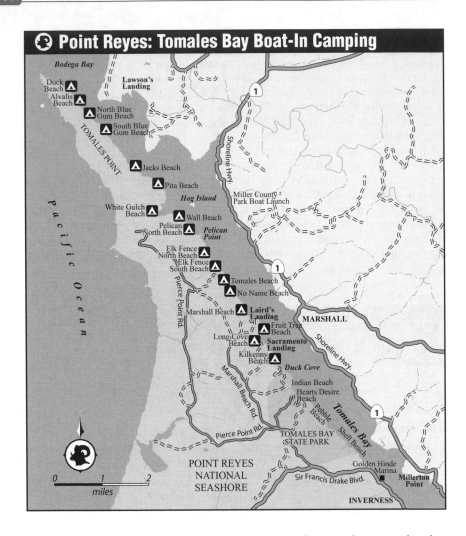

Point Reyes: Tomales Bay Boat-In Camping

Wind is common, however, and can quickly turn placid waters into roiling whitecaps, especially when cold fog piles up over Point Reyes and hot conditions prevail inland; the sharp temperature difference often creates intense localized winds. Paddlers can hug the shoreline for safety and shelter, and should always be on watch for changing conditions.

The trip begins from Tomales Bay State Park and heads north along the western edge of Tomales Bay, passing numerous designated camping beaches along the way. Water is *not* available; bring as much as you'll need. Tides strongly influence currents in Tomales Bay. Note the tide times to take advantage of incoming and outgoing currents, which can significantly aid your progression. Note that there is roughly a one-hour delay between posted tide times for the mouth of Tomales Bay and points midway down the bay. Currents and exposure become more severe as you approach the bay entrance north of White Gulch Beach; paddling experience and caution are recommended.

Trail Camps

There are more than **15 designated beaches** for camping, stretching from just north of Tomales Bay State Park to the mouth of Tomales Bay, a distance of more than 10 miles. This trip visits 12 of them but does not include the farthest beaches near the bay mouth, which require good paddling experience to reach safely. Some beaches provide outhouses, while others do not. Most paddlers camp directly on the sand; a few locations offer more shelter in nearby woods. All overnight sites are located within Point Reyes National Seashore; *camping on state park land is prohibited.*

Camping is by permit only. Reservations may be made up to three months in advance (to the day) by calling (415) 663-8054, 9 a.m.–2 p.m. Monday through Friday. Reservations can also be made in person at the Bear Valley Visitor Center during open hours or by fax (download the appropriate form at **www.nps.gov/pore**). Except for the busiest weekends, boat-in sites are usually available; walk-in registration is normally possible for same-day departures.

Permits cost $15 per night for 1–6 people, $30 per night for 7–14 people, and $40 per night for 15–25 people. Permits must be obtained from the Bear Valley Visitor Center prior to leaving on your trip. It is open 9 a.m.–5 p.m. weekdays, and 8 a.m.–5 p.m. weekends and holidays. After-hours pick-up is allowed—permits are placed in a

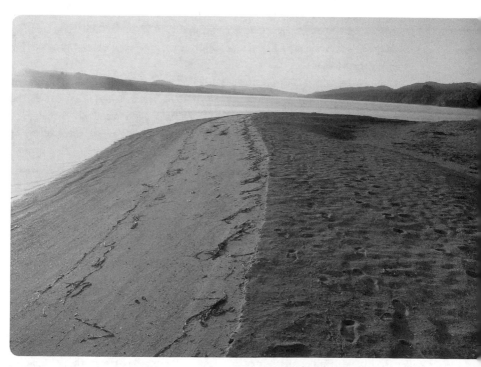

Looking south from Fruit Tree Beach

HUMAN HISTORY OF POINT REYES

Once the site of more than 100 Coast Miwok Indian villages, the Point Reyes peninsula was conquered by the Spanish by the early 19th century. Introduced diseases devastated the indigenous population. Many left the area for nearby Mission San Rafael (established in 1817), further reducing their numbers. Left to fend for themselves following the secularization of the missions in the 1830s, most remaining Miwok died.

Following the 1821 overthrow of its Spanish governors, Mexico began giving out massive land grants. Several large parcels on Point Reyes peninsula were distributed, but became the subject of controversy because of loosely defined property boundaries. Once the U.S. acquired California in the late 1840s, a long series of complicated legal battles eventually put the entire peninsula in the hands of just three (American) men—Oscar and James Shafter, and Charles Webb Howard. The three quickly began leasing their land to dairy farmers. Soon these ranches were producing high-quality butter for shipment to San Francisco. In the 1860s, ranches were identified by the letters of the alphabet. Starting with A Ranch by the Point Reyes lighthouse, the ranches progressed clockwise around the peninsula to Z Ranch on Mt. Wittenberg.

After World War II, local conservationists began lobbying for the creation of a national park. On September 13, 1962, President John F. Kennedy signed the bill creating the national seashore and authorizing acquisition of 53,000 acres. Over the ensuing decade, the land was slowly acquired, though existing ranches continued operation under long-term leases.

The wilderness area of the seashore was designated in 1976. Ranch structures were torn down, their legacy left in the network of roads and trails that crisscross the wilderness area. In 1985 the wilderness was named for Congressman Phillip Burton, a long-time representative from San Francisco who worked hard to expand the acreage in the national park system.

wooden box by the information board in front of the visitor center.

Getting There

You'll first need to visit the Bear Valley Visitor Center to pick up your permit. Head to the small town of Olema on Highway 1. From the intersection of Highway 1 and Sir Francis Drake Boulevard, proceed north on Highway 1 and make an immediate left on Bear Valley Road. In 0.5 mile, turn left again to reach the visitor center.

To reach the put-in, take Bear Valley Road 2 miles north of the visitor center and proceed north on Sir Francis Drake Boulevard for 5.7 miles to Pierce Point Road; you pass Golden Hinde Inn and Marina in 4.1 miles, another possible launch site described below. Turn right on Pierce Point Road and continue 1.2 miles to the turnoff for Hearts Desire Beach in Tomales Bay State Park. Follow the turnoff to its end, where a day-use parking area (fee charged) is available. From here, you

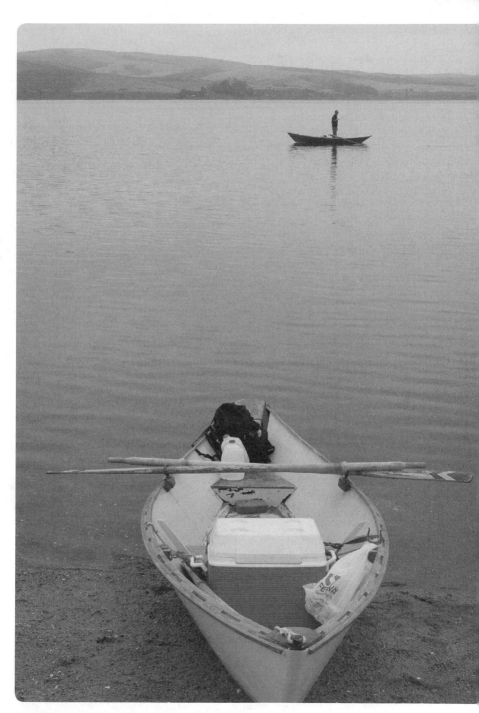

The wildlife and waters of Tomales Bay await your visit.

will need to carry your boat approximately 100 yards to the beach and launch site; there is *not* a boat ramp.

Overnight parking is prohibited in Tomales Bay State Park. If possible, arrange for a drop-off. If you need to leave your vehicle overnight, the closest option is Golden Hinde Inn and Marina, 4 road miles away from the put-in site. You can also launch here (fee charged), which adds 3 miles to your overall paddling journey.

Several launch sites are also available on the east side of the bay, including Millerton Point, Miller County Park, and Lawson's Landing. These options all require you to cross the bay, however, adding additional exposure to your journey if conditions are rough.

Boating It

Wildlife is prolific in Tomales Bay. Over the course of your journey, watch for the following: harbor seals, sea lions, bat rays, coyotes, raccoons, tule elk, ospreys, red-tailed hawks, snowy egrets, great blue herons, brown and white pelicans, loons, cormorants, quail, kingfishers, and owls. At night, listen for the breathing of seals and sea lions as they come up for air.

The San Andreas Fault underlies Tomales Bay, grinding the rocks along the fault into easily eroded sediment and creating the deep trough of the bay. The linear fault continues northwest under the bay entrance and southwest through distinctive Inverness Valley.

Get on the water and head north from Hearts Desire Beach, avoiding the designated swimming area on your way to nearby Indian Beach (0.4). Here several tepeelike structures recreate a type of shelter used by the Miwok Indians, the region's original inhabitants. A pleasant 0.5-mile nature trail connects Indian Beach with Hearts

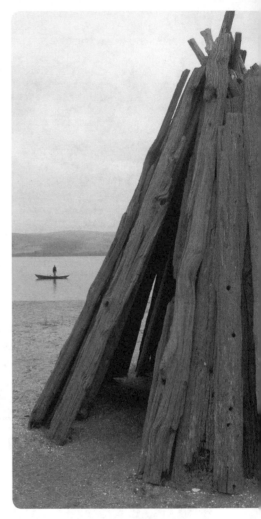

Reconstructed Miwok shelter at Indian Beach

Desire Beach, passing through a lush mixed-evergreen forest of Douglas-fir, huckleberry, and abundant ferns.

Mixed-evergreen woods also cloak the adjacent hillsides as you continue north, including Monterey pine, bay trees, and alder. Windswept specimens indicate the area's predominant northwest winds. You pass private Duck Cove (1.0), where a collection of small dinghies sit near several buildings and homes. You next float past Kilkenny Beach (1.2), the first available camping option. It is low on wilderness feel, however—an old red building sits next to the small sandy strip and power and telephone lines cross the area.

Continuing, you pass private Sacramento Landing to reach Long Cove and its small beach (1.8), which is tucked deeply into the surrounding headlands and offers good shelter from the wind. Next up is diminutive Fruit Tree Beach (2.1), a nice sandy strand mostly covered at high tide. It offers excellent views of the bay and features several granite outcrops along the edges of the beach.

Bull kelp begins to appear as you proceed north along the rocky headlands and bluffs to Laird's Landing (2.5), where several unoccupied buildings nestle in the trees. Camping is *not* allowed here, though an enticing rope swing may tempt you to stop. Just ahead is popular Marshall Beach (2.7), the northernmost beach accessible by trail along Point Reyes' eastern flanks; a wide fire road provides inland access. Tall Monterey cypresses loom over the broad strand, shading several grassy campsites. A smaller spit of sand at the north end of the beach provides another nice camping option. Outhouses are available.

Your next destination is No Name Beach (3.3), a small beach surrounded by dense willow thickets that indicate the approaching transition from woodlands to more open coastal headlands. The water is shallow here; you may have difficulty landing at low tide. Just beyond is Tomales Beach (3.6), a long curving stretch of sand with outhouses and an abundance of good campsites. A small ridge behind the beach provides good views north to Elk Fence South and North beaches, your next destina-

tions. You can also pick out Pelican Point, protruding from the western shore in front of Hog Island.

Rounding a corner, you encounter narrow Elk Fence South Beach (3.9) tucked in a shallow cove; an ephemeral stream flows in through thick willows. North around the next small point is Elk Fence North Beach (4.2), a thin beach with little sand at high tide. Open rolling hills rise behind it, providing good access for wandering the headlands.

The area's namesake fence, separating the seashore's herd of tule elk from roaming cattle, can be spotted to the south. Originally native to the area, tule elk were reintroduced in 1978 by the National Park Service. Today they number in the hundreds and can often be spotted roaming the open headlands of Tomales Point beyond this point.

The next landmark north is Pelican Point (4.8), a sand spit that extends as an underwater shoal to a prominent red navigation post. Pelican Point is closed to visitors to protect wildlife habitat—do *not* land. Pelican North Beach (5.1), on the other hand, invites you to step onto its sheltered sands. An adjacent grove of eucalyptus shades a thin water source, and good campsites dot the area.

You pass Wall Beach (5.4) on your continuing journey north, a tiny strand that all but disappears at high tide. Much better is White Gulch Beach (6.0), located in a large, idyllic cove and named for the prominent white rock outcrops. Views of Tomales Bay diminish as you enter the cove, which provides a self-contained world of wild California. Rolling hills tracked with tule elk game trails surround the area, providing extensive opportunities to wander this wild place. Sandy beach is in short supply for camping, though abundant grassy areas serve as potential campsites. Sweeping views of the landscape increase as you head upslope from water's edge.

Past White Gulch Beach, currents and wind become stronger as you approach the bay entrance. Solid paddling experience and good weather conditions are recommended if you wish to continue. Pita Beach (6.5) is the next option, tucked into the broad headlands that hem White Gulch in to the north. It offers campers a pleasant sandy beach and good shelter from northwest wind. Beyond Pita Beach is Jacks Beach (7.2), then three camping options along the bay entrance: North

Blue Gum Beach (8.8), Alvalis Beach (9.2), and Duck Beach (9.5). Adventure and discovery await intrepid paddlers in these wild places, which sit at the nexus of ocean, bay, land, wind, and tide.

Giving Back

The **Point Reyes National Seashore Association** works to preserve the extraordinary wilderness of Point Reyes and to educate the public about the environment. Contact the association or learn more at (415) 663-1200 or **www.ptreyes.org**.

9 Austin Creek State Recreation Area

RATINGS	Scenery **7** Difficulty **6** Solitude **8**
ROUND-TRIP DISTANCE	6.4 to 10.5 miles, depending on route
ELEVATION GAIN/LOSS	+1,900'/–1,900' to +2,200'/–2,200', depending on route
OPTIONAL MAP	*Austin Creek State Recreation Area Map* by California State Parks
BEST TIMES	March through November
AGENCY	Austin Creek State Recreation Area, California State Parks, (707) 869-2015, **www.parks.ca.gov**
PERMIT	Contact Armstrong Redwoods State Reserve and Austin Creek State Recreation Area, 17000 Armstrong Woods Rd., Guerneville, CA 95446, (707) 869-2015, **www.parks.ca.gov**. The visitor center, (707) 869-2958, is open 11 a.m.–3 p.m. daily, with longer hours in the summer. The park entrance station is open approximately 8 a.m.–sunset daily.

Highlights

A hidden, wild world lurks in the rumpled Coast Range north of the Russian River. Here you will find a diverse natural world of oak woodlands, redwood groves, far-reaching vistas, and fantastic spring wildflowers, all tucked deep within secluded canyons. To get to the

trailhead, you must drive a thrilling, one-lane road that first passes beneath the gigantic old-growth redwoods of Armstrong Redwoods State Reserve before climbing more than 1,000 feet at a 12-percent grade to dead-end atop a ridge with spectacular views.

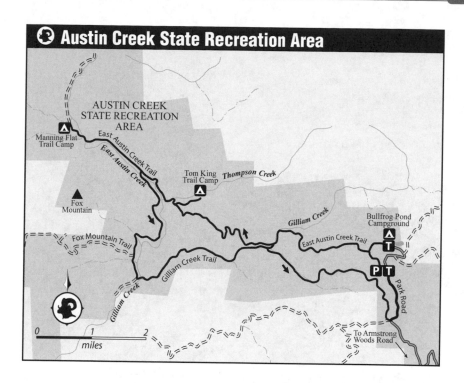

⊙ Austin Creek State Recreation Area

Hike Overview

The trail descends steeply from ridgeline to lush valley bottom, visiting four mellifluous streams, two different trail camps, and a wide diversity of ecosystems. The full 10.5-mile loop journey along East Austin Creek and Gilliam Creek trails to Manning Flat Trail Camp is described below, though shorter trips are possible. The quickest overnight excursion is the 6.4-mile out-and-back journey to Tom King Trail Camp on East Austin Creek Trail. Several other semiloops that use only portions of Gilliam Creek Trail are also possible. East Austin Creek Trail is a broad service road; Gilliam Creek Trail is single-track and open to hikers and equestrians only.

Note that in recent years the park has closed the trail camps from December through June due to budget cuts. Always check in advance before planning a trip here.

Trail Camps

Two trail camps are available for overnight use: Manning Flat and Tom King. **Tom King** is closest to the trailhead (3.2 miles one way) and located at the end of a 0.3-mile spur trail. There is only one site at Tom King, located beneath buckeye and bay trees. Gurgling Thompson Creek flows alongside; a few redwoods grow in the streambed.

In the far western corner of the park, **Manning Flat** features two well-spaced sites beneath the shady boughs of Douglas-fir and bay trees near broad East Austin Creek. You must ford the bridgeless stream to reach Manning Flat, a potential challenge during the

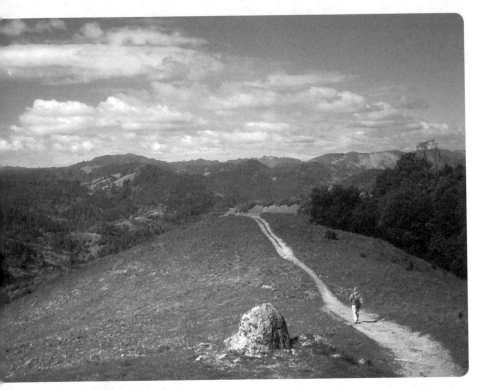

Deep in the Coast Range wild

rainy season. Potable water, picnic tables, fire rings, and restrooms are provided at both trail camps. Campfires are not allowed during fire season (typically late July through October).

Trail camps are available on a first-come, first-served basis, and all arriving backpackers must obtain a backcountry permit on the day of their trip. (You can call ahead for availability.) Permits can only be obtained from the park entry kiosk or from an on-duty park ranger. The volunteer-staffed Armstrong Redwoods visitor center (see below) may be able to help locate a ranger. There is a fee of $25 per site, and a maximum capacity of 8 people per site. Trail camps are regularly used

and fill most weekends year-round, but less on weekdays. Bullfrog Pond Campground (22 first-come, first-served sites) is adjacent to the trailhead and an option for a Friday arrival and Saturday departure to a trail camp.

Getting There

Take either Highway 116 or River Road west from Highway 101 to Guerneville and turn north on Armstrong Woods Road, located 0.1 mile west of the Russian River Bridge. In 2.5 miles you reach the Armstrong Redwoods park entrance and visitor center. A thrilling 2.5 miles later you reach the East Austin Creek Trailhead at Vista Point. This final 2.5 miles of road is narrow and twisting, with several steep (12-percent grade) 5 mile-per-hour hairpin turns. Vehicles longer than 20 feet are *not* permitted. Park staff will advise you on where to park your vehicle overnight.

Hiking It

The region's topography is severe—a world of closely packed ridges rising more than 1,000 feet above narrow canyons barely 200 feet above sea level. The San Andreas Fault slices the coastal margin less than 10 miles away, slowly moving land west of the fault, such as nearby Bodega Head, north along the edge of California. While the majority of fault motion occurs directly along the San Andreas itself, some of the force is translated inland; nearby lands are riddled with smaller faults and have thus been sheared, compressed, and squeezed upward. The high rainfall of the area has dissected and eroded the folded landscape into the convoluted topography present today.

Within this tortured geography, Austin Creek State Recreation Area straddles an ecological divide between coastal redwood forest and drier oak woodland. Only 10 miles from the ocean, yet guarded from summer fog by several intervening ridges, the area receives significant precipitation (more than 50 inches) in the winter months yet bakes during the summer in temperatures that can approach 100°F. The results are perennial streams in narrow canyons lined with ferns, Douglas-fir, and redwoods; exposed hills of open grasslands dotted with twisting oaks and spring wildflowers; slopes with southern exposures cloaked with chaparral; and surprising pockets of redwood forest on shady north-facing slopes. Sudden oak death has been identified in the park—please take precautions against spreading this blight to other areas (see page 20 for more information).

From the trailhead (0.0/1,400'), savor the sweeping view across the rolling terrain. Your journey down wide East Austin Creek Trail passes through a variety of ecosystems: Sun-exposed west-facing slopes feature coyote brush, manzanita, and several species of oak—coast, Oregon, and black; the moist shelter of nearby gullies nourishes bay trees, willow, buckeye, and poison oak; and shady north- and east-facing slopes support water-loving Douglas-fir and redwoods.

Descending on East Austin Creek Trail, you soon pass a single-track spur trail on the right, which comes from lower Bullfrog Pond Campground (0.2/1,150'). Continue the steep drop on a hillside regularly rooted by wild pigs and seasonally flushed with wildflowers. Baby blue eyes, shooting stars, and brodiaea are particularly abundant. Numerous rock outcrops of greenstone also are present, a component of the Franciscan Formation (see "Bay Area Geology," page 13). Near canyon bottom, the trail curves right and descends into a thickening mixed-evergreen forest. You briefly travel above crystalline Gilliam Creek, then reach it near a bridge and junction for the short spur trail that leads to nearby Gilliam Creek Trail (1.5/340').Those fortunate to be here in March may witness orange-bellied newts congregating by the dozens to mate in these waters.

Cross the bridge over Gilliam Creek and continue on wide East Austin Creek Trail as it climbs briefly up a small, unnamed drainage brimming with giant chain ferns, bigleaf maple, and peeling madrone. You then climb above it all to open oak hillsides with exceptional views. The small linear valley of Thompson Creek is visible to the north (where Tom King Trail Camp resides) and the deep drainage of East Austin Creek twists southwest toward the Russian River. After cresting near coast live oaks (2.5/750'), descend to the junction with Tom King Trail (2.9/450'). If you're camping at Tom King, or just looking for an idyllic picnic spot, turn right here and proceed a gentle 0.3 mile to camp at trail's end.

To continue to Manning Flat Trail Camp, remain on East Austin Creek Trail as it switchbacks twice and crosses Thompson Creek. Large, old-growth redwoods appear across the stream as the wide trail now parallels East Austin Creek to reach the junction (3.5/190') with Gilliam Creek Trail. Continue on East Austin Creek Trail to reach camp 0.7 mile beyond the junction; the sites are immediately past the unbridged creek crossing.

Back at the trail junction (3.5/190'), ford East Austin Creek on Gilliam Creek Trail to enter shadier east-facing slopes covered by an understory of sword, wood, and maidenhair ferns. Climbing briefly, the trail winds well above the rushing stream and its narrow canyon before descending again to reach Fox Mountain Trail on the right (4.6/290'). Continue straight, then bear left, and descend the single-track trail to reach the confluence of East Austin and Gilliam creeks. Ford East Austin Creek to reach an old trail campsite (4.9/240'), now a large grassy field near the creek.

The trail next winds through a narrow canyon beneath shady bay trees, oaks, buckeye, bigleaf maple, and Douglas-fir. You briefly climb a short distance above the creek, then descend to cross and recross it nine times over the next mile. The stream crossings are not always obvious (only a few are signed), but the trail is apparent; if you find yourself on a disappearing track, retrace your steps. At Schoolhouse Creek you encounter the junction for a short connector to East Austin Creek Trail (6.5/360'). Although that route provides the most direct route back to the trailhead, you enjoy more variety and views straight on Gilliam Creek Trail.

Continuing on Gilliam Creek Trail, cross the creek three more times before beginning a steep climb along a small feeder creek to an open, oak-studded ridge. Manzanita, toyon, and chamise line the trail as it steadily ascends the ridgeline before leveling and banking right to traverse the upper Schoolhouse Creek drainage (passing through several nice redwood groves en route). The trail alternately contours gently and ascends steeply to reach the junction with East Ridge Trail and the park road (8.5/1,300'). Savor the beautiful vistas one last time as you bear left (north) and hike along the park road to return to the trailhead (9.1/1,400').

Giving Back

Stewards of the Coast and Redwoods is a nonprofit group that works in partnership with California State Parks to protect and interpret the natural and cultural resources of the Russian River and Sonoma Coast districts. Contact the group at P.O. Box 2, Duncan Mills, CA 95430, or (707) 869-9177, or learn more at **www.stewardsofthecoastand redwoods.org.**

Santa Cruz Mountains

Redwood forest blankets the Santa Cruz Mountains with a sylvan world unlike any other on Earth. Come experience the majesty of these mighty trees, including extensive stands of old-growth hundreds of years old. A range of adjoining ecosystems, unusual geology, and distant views add to the region's remarkable backpacking opportunities.

A rugged, ridge-lined landscape deeply incised by a multitude of creeks, the geography of the Santa Cruz Mountains is largely defined by the axis of long, northwest-trending Skyline Ridge. Stretching more than 50 miles from near Gilroy to Highway 92 above Half Moon Bay, it rises some 3,000 feet and separates the developed Bay Area from the wild heart of these mountains. West of Skyline Ridge, a multitude of creeks and rivers tumble toward the ocean, the largest of which are (from north to south) Pescadero Creek, Waddell Creek, and the San Lorenzo River.

Most of the Santa Cruz Mountains and its protected parklands are located along the west side of Skyline Ridge. In the heart of the mountains lies a large complex of contiguous and interconnected parks centered around the Pescadero and Waddell creek drainages—Sam McDonald, Memorial, and Pescadero Creek county parks and Portola Redwoods, Butano, Castle Rock, and Big Basin Redwoods state parks. With the exception of Butano, all of these parks either border each other or are connected via a network of trails. With more than 10 backcountry trail camps in this complex, opportunities for overnight adventures among the redwoods are extensive.

10 Monte Bello Open Space Preserve Loop

RATINGS	Scenery **5** Difficulty **2** Solitude **5**
ROUND-TRIP DISTANCE	5.0 miles
ELEVATION GAIN	+1,200'/–1,200'
OPTIONAL MAP	*Monte Bello Open Space Preserve Map* by Midpeninsula Regional Open Space District
BEST TIMES	Year-round
AGENCY	Midpeninsula Regional Open Space District, (650) 691-1200, **www.openspace.org**
PERMIT	Trail camp reservations are required. Call MROSD during office hours (8:30 a.m.–5 p.m.) There is a fee of $2 per person.

Highlights

Monte Bello lulls in more ways than one. A single-track interpretive nature trail winds along the headwaters of Stevens Creek. A steady climb rises above the deep crease formed by the grinding San Andreas Fault. A trail camp awaits atop distinct Black Mountain (2,800'). Savory, ever-changing views peer into a hidden valley and beyond. *Monte Bello, que bello.*

Hike Overview

This short loop atop Monte Bello Ridge is an easy adventure along narrow trails and broad fire roads. Tucked in a narrow crease immediately east of the long axis of Skyline Ridge and Highway 35, this hike visits the only trail camp on the eastern slopes of the Santa Cruz Mountains. The park is quiet and secluded, remarkable given its proximity to downtown Cupertino and Silicon Valley (only 8 miles away).

The hike is described counterclockwise, beginning along educational Stevens Creek Nature Trail, which makes for a longer, more informative hike in and an easier hike out. The hike can be completed year-round, though trails above Stevens Creek corridor are exposed and hot in summer. (The trail camp is pleasantly shaded.) Spring wildflowers are excellent. *Dogs are prohibited.*

Trail Camp

Black Mountain Trail Camp is situated a quarter mile from the summit of Black Mountain at an elevation of 2,700 feet. It consists of four small sites (maximum four people per site) and one group site (maximum 24). The sites are stacked close together, but usage is light and the camp is seldom full. For such a pristine-feeling park, the trail camp and surrounding area are surprisingly developed—radio towers dot the summit, the bathroom is illuminated at night, and phone and power cables stretch overhead. Good views to the west are available nearby, but views of the often hazy South Bay are mostly obscured by vegetation. Nonpotable water (bring a filter or boil it) and food

⊙ Monte Bello Open Space Preserve Loop

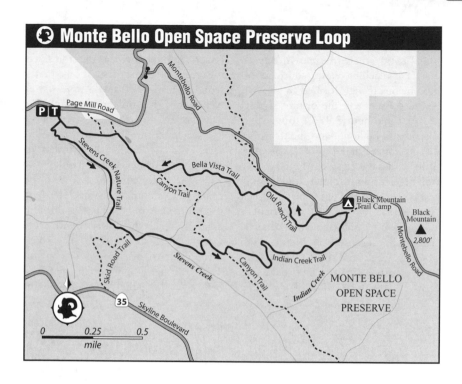

lockers are provided. *Campfires are prohibited.*

Getting There

Take Interstate 280 to the Page Mill Road exit west of Palo Alto. Follow Page Mill Road west for 7 miles to reach the main entrance and parking area on the left. Alternatively, take Highway 35 for 7 miles south of the junction of Highways 84 and 35, then bear left (east) on Page Mill Road and proceed 1.5 miles to the main entrance on the right.

Hiking It

Before you begin, take a moment to appreciate this special preserve. Taller than neighboring Skyline Ridge to the west, Monte Bello Ridge is an anomalous rise on the eastern slopes of the Santa Cruz Mountains. At its base,

sandwiched between the two steep ridges, the San Andreas Fault slices across the landscape and pulverizes the rock found along its trace. Stevens Creek, flowing eastward to enter the San Francisco Bay near Mountain View, easily cut through this loose material to carve a narrow, secluded canyon more than a thousand feet deep. The cool depths provide moisture and shelter for a mixed-evergreen forest more typical of regions farther west in the Santa Cruz Mountains, while the west-facing slopes of Monte Bello Ridge quickly transition to dry oak woodland, open grassland, and chaparral communities more common farther inland. Wildlife is abundant and varied as well—deer, newts, tarantulas, raptors, owls, lizards, frogs, coyotes, and bobcats all make the preserve their home.

The hike begins by the information sign at the trailhead parking lot (0.0/2,230'), where free maps are available. Far-reaching views south reveal the obvious trough formed by the San Andreas Fault. On the distant skyline are Mt. Umunhum (3,486'), topped by a rectangular building, and slightly more distant Loma Prieta (3,806'), epicenter of its namesake 1989 earthquake. The trail descends immediately and quickly reaches the junction with Stevens Creek Nature Trail (0.1/2,200'). Bear right.

Interpretive signs elucidate natural features as Stevens Creek Nature Trail descends via several short switchbacks. Bay, madrone, canyon live oak, and ferns fill the lush alley of dribbling Stevens Creek as the trail follows its drainage. Coast live oak and Douglas-fir soon join the forest as the trail skirts the creek and then crosses it on a pretty wooden bridge. Tanoak appears as well before the trail briefly climbs 30 feet above the increasingly steep gully.

Reaching the junction with Skid Road Trail (1.2/1,800'), bear left to remain on Stevens Creek Trail. Now wider, it briefly continues close to the creek before contouring upslope past some large firs and then passes through a gate to reach the junction with wide Canyon Trail (1.8/1,920'). The route turns right to briefly follow Canyon Trail through some open clearings before reaching the junction with In-

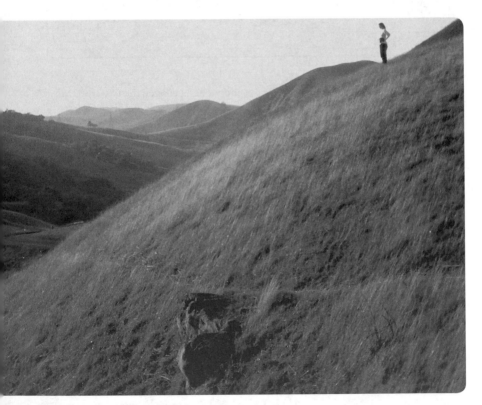

A hiker looks into Monte Bello Open Space Preserve.

dian Creek Trail (2.0/1,970'). Head left toward Backpack Camp on Indian Creek Trail as Canyon Trail continues its journey downstream.

Buckeye, coyote brush, large twisting valley oaks, toyon, coffee berry, and yerba santa all appear on the drier, more exposed slopes as the trail steadily climbs, and large amounts of chamise grow closer to the top. Increasingly good views open up until the trail encounters the posted junction for the trail camp (3.0/2,700'). The antenna-clad summit of Black Mountain is a short 0.4 mile ahead, but bear left instead to reach the campsites. The trail camp is located on the same site as the original buildings of Black Mountain Ranch, torn down following the acquisition of this property by MROSD in 1978. An interpretive placard providing further details can be found nearby, along with an active seismic monitoring station and views of distant Mt. Tamalpais.

To return to the trailhead, follow the road from camp northwest along the ridge, then go left at the junction with Old Ranch Trail (3.2/2,660'). Go left again at the junction with Bella Vista Trail (3.6/2,540'). Some of the farthest reaching views yet can be enjoyed along this section: Mt. Tamalpais in Marin, Mt. Diablo in the East Bay, and the Dumbarton Bridge in the South Bay. Passing above several thin, oak-choked gullies, Bella Vista Trail passes numerous buckeyes as it slowly descends to Canyon Trail (4.4/2,130'). Turn right on Canyon Trail and pass a small, marshy sag pond on the right filled with cattails. Sag ponds are common along the San Andreas Fault and are formed as fault motion pulls apart the ground to form small depressions. Bear left shortly before Canyon Trail reaches Page Mill Road (4.6/2,100'), and follow signs for the single-track Nature Trail Return Loop. Many use trails crisscross this area before the trail rejoins the initial junction below the parking lot (5.0/2,230').

Giving Back

The **Midpeninsula Regional Open Space District** is a nonprofit that purchases, permanently protects, and restores lands forming a regional open space greenbelt along the San Francisco peninsula, from Saratoga to Half Moon Bay. Learn more and donate online at **www.openspace.org**.

11 Butano State Park Loop

RATINGS	Scenery **5** Difficulty **4** Solitude **7**
ROUND-TRIP DISTANCE	9.8 miles
ELEVATION GAIN/LOSS	+2,100'/–2,100'
OPTIONAL MAP	*Butano State Park Map* by California State Parks
BEST TIMES	Year-round
AGENCY	Butano State Park, (650) 879-2040, **www.parks.ca.gov**
PERMIT	A first-come, first-served trail camp permit is required. Register at the park entrance station.

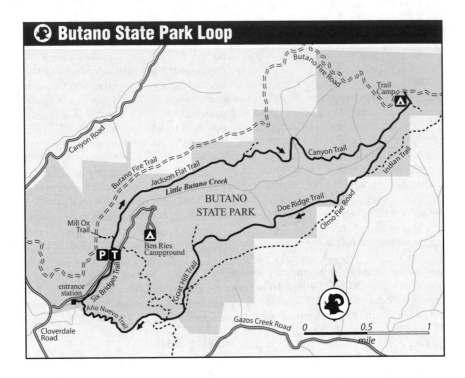

Butano State Park Loop

Highlights

Little Butano Creek slices westward in a narrow defile almost completely protected within Butano (BOO-tah-no) State Park. Less than 4 miles long yet brimming with ecological diversity, the canyon contains an isolated and diverse world representative of the entire region. A lightly used trail camp and a loop hike almost exclusively on single-track make this an alluring trip.

Hike Overview

The hike travels on seven different trails to loop clockwise around the canyon. It can be completed in either direction, but hiking counterclockwise necessitates a steep climb of nearly 1,000 feet (with full packs) at the start of the adventure. Otherwise the elevation gain is significant but generally

gradual. Spring and fall offer the most ideal combination of good weather and light crowds. Summer is foggy and more crowded. Winter and early spring are typically rainy, but the rewards are an explosion of fascinating fungi, clambering newts, and the opportunity to discover the bloom of the purple calypso orchid. *Bikes and dogs are prohibited.*

Trail Camps

Seven primitive sites are located at the ridgeline headwaters of Little Butano Creek in a thick canopy of young redwood forest. They consist of small clearings with very basic chairs and tables made of planks and logs. An outhouse is located nearby, but picnic tables and food lockers are not provided. Campfires are not permitted and water is not available within camp—

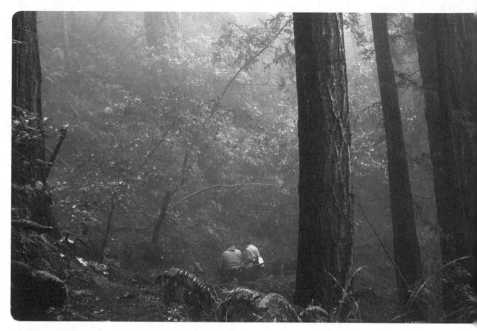

Doe Ridge Trail

the closest source is perennial Little Butano Creek a half mile away. Open year-round, the trail camp receives light use and offers excellent privacy. All sites are first-come, first-served, and the seldom-visited trail camp reportedly never fills. There is a maximum of six people per site. Register at the park entrance station upon arrival. Sites cost $10 per night.

Getting There

From the north, take Highway 1 south of Half Moon Bay for 16 miles to Pescadero Road and turn left. In 2.5 miles, turn right on Cloverdale Road and proceed 4 miles to the park entrance on the left. Approaching from Santa Cruz, take Highway 1 north of Davenport for 14 miles and turn right on Gazos Creek Road, located immediately north of the Beach House gas

station. Follow Gazos Creek Road for 2 miles, turn left on Cloverdale Road, and follow the narrow twisting road for 1 mile to the park entrance on the right. The trailhead at Mill Ox Trail is a half mile past the entrance station by a large turnout. Overnight users can park their car in any day-use parking lot.

Hiking It

From the trailhead (0.0/230'), begin on Mill Ox Trail as it crosses Little Butano Creek and quickly climbs northeast to reach the junction with Jackson Flat Trail (0.2/430'). The route initially weaves through redwoods, Douglas-fir, tanoak, and huckleberry bushes; big-leaf maple, twisting madrone, the soft leaves of hazel, and sword and wood fern also appear intermittently. Turn right on Jackson Flat Trail to begin a gradual rising traverse that runs along the moisture divide between a damp redwood forest (a few large old-growth trees can be spotted) and a drier mixed-evergreen forest.

Bear right onto Canyon Trail (1.7/800') at the junction as Jackson Flat Trail curves left, and continue through thick redwood forest. Soon the woods change to a shorter forest of canyon live oak and madrone, and then abruptly transform into an entirely different ecosystem as the trail crosses the threshold of the Santa Margarita Formation. Here xeric sandstone, poor in water and organic material, attracts species better adapted to these harsh conditions. Knobcone pine proliferates here, a spindly conifer with namesake cones that grow everywhere (including on branches and trunks).

Knobcone pines survive through serotiny—their cones open only from the heat of wildfires. In an environment where fire frequency is every 20 to 40 years, this successful strategy populates the newly charred, nutrient-rich soil with a massive, sudden influx of seeds. Joining knobcone pines are other members of the chaparral community: manzanita, golden chinquapin (look under the leaves), toyon berry, scrub oak (the mini-oak shrub), and chamise—one of the most common members of the driest chaparral communities.

As the trail winds through this open community, outstanding views reveal the depth of this diminutive canyon, just one of many to explore in the Santa Cruz Mountains. Next the trail banks left into a small tributary canyon and narrows, descending on steep slopes to cross a seasonally rushing creek (note the bigleaf maples and change of ecosystem as moisture again increases). Then it climbs back out via several switchbacks to rejoin the Santa

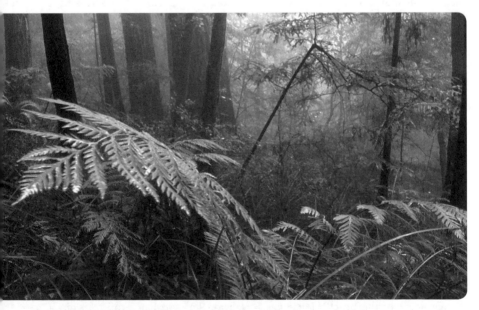

Giant chain ferns grow in the redwood forest understory.

Margarita Formation and accompanying views and flora.

Contouring around several small drainages, the trail returns to thick forest and reaches the posted junction for the trail camp (3.7/1,200'). To reach the trail camp, bear left and head steeply uphill along the narrow overgrown trail to reach a junction with an unnamed fire road (4.2/1,460') and turn left (uphill). The sites are well spread out to the left of the fire road between here and nearby Butano Fire Road. Ray Linder Memorial Trail, dedicated to a former park ranger, is nearby.

To begin the journey home, return to the junction with Canyon Trail (4.7/1,200') and continue briefly up-canyon before the trail crosses young Little Butano Creek and soon reaches Olmo Fire Road (5.2/1,240'). Turn right. For the next 0.4 mile, the route follows Olmo Fire Road through private property owned by Ainsley Family Tree Farm. Please respect property rights and stay on the road as it descends to reach the posted junction with Doe Ridge Trail on the right (5.5/1,050'). Along the way, enjoy looking south into intriguing Gazos Creek drainage, the only views of the hike beyond Little Butano Creek.

The route turns right onto single-track Doe Ridge Trail and passes through one of its most idyllic stretches—level, nicely contoured, and beneath old-growth redwoods (there are 315 acres of old-growth redwood forest protected within the park). At the junction with Goat Hill Trail (7.0/840'), turn left and continue through a thick Douglas-fir forest recovering from recent logging. Goat Hill Trail passes a spur trail on the left (7.5/900') leading to adjacent Olmo Fire Road, and then another spur a short distance later

(7.6/920'). From here, Goat Hill Trail continues downhill to the right toward the campground and offers a more direct and less strenuous route back to trailhead—just follow the road from the campground. (It also necessitates dealing with vehicles and pavement.)

To avoid the campground and road area and maximize single-track hiking, return to Olmo Fire Road and bear right to reach the junction on the left for Año Nuevo Trail (8.0/1,060'). This is your last chance to choose the easier route to the trailhead—Olmo Fire Road also connects with the campground and road. Otherwise bear left on Año Nuevo Trail and contour briefly along a forested ridge of Douglas-fir. The trail banks right and down-canyon, then drops directly on switchbacks. The foliage becomes thick with elderberry and blackberry as airy views of the canyon's end and the entrance station appear. At the bottom (9.3/220'), bear right at the bridge on Six Bridges Trail and proceed along the banks of Little Butano Creek to return to the trailhead. Enjoy the euphonious flow of this peaceful stream as you wind back and forth along level ground to end your journey (9.8/230').

Giving Back

Sempervirens Fund is a nonprofit land conservancy dedicated to preserving, expanding, and linking parklands in the Santa Cruz Mountains. Contact the group or learn more at (650) 949-1453 or **www.sempervirens.org**.

The nonprofit **San Mateo Coast Natural History Association** works to maintain and enhance California State Parks along the San Mateo Coast, including Butano State Park. Contact the association or learn more at (650) 345-2001 or **www.sanmateocoastnha.org**.

12 Pescadero Creek County Park Loop

RATINGS	Scenery **6** Difficulty **4** Solitude **8**
ROUND-TRIP DISTANCE	10.5 miles
ELEVATION GAIN/LOSS	+1,500'/–1,500'
OPTIONAL MAP	*Pescadero Creek County Park Map* by San Mateo County Parks
BEST TIMES	Year-round
AGENCY	Sam McDonald and Pescadero Creek county parks; both are managed from Memorial County Park, (650) 879-0238; San Mateo County Parks and Recreation Division, (650) 363-4020, **www.eparks.net**
PERMIT	Shaw Flat Trail Camp is first-come, first-served. Register at the Memorial County Park entrance station when it is staffed.

Highlights

Deep and secluded, pocketed with untouched redwood groves and lined with gurgling streams, Pescadero Creek County Park covers more than 6,000 acres in the heart of the Santa Cruz Mountains. Amid it all hides Shaw Flat Trail Camp, a remote backcountry destination accessed via the tall ridgelines and redwoods of Sam McDonald County Park.

Hike Overview

This loop hike provides big-picture views of the area, descending from open ridgetop to lush redwood-filled canyon. Traversing first along a ridgeline above the Pescadero Creek drainage, the route then loops in and out of the canyon on impressive single-track Brook Trail Loop, reaching the trail camp in the valley bottom at the midpoint of the hike.

Trail Camp

Shaw Flat Trail Camp perches 100 feet above hidden Pescadero Creek and consists of several sites spread beneath the branches of second-growth redwood forest. Potable water is *not* provided, but nearby Pescadero Creek can be accessed a quarter mile away. A few picnic tables are scattered among the sites and an outhouse is available. The camp is open year-round and conditions are usually the same at all times—cool and damp. The rainy season entails more cold and wet, but it also brings an explosion of fungi and migrating newts. *Campfires and dogs are prohibited.*

Getting There

Take Highway 84 to Pescadero Road, 1 mile east of the small town of La Honda. Follow Pescadero Road south for 1.5 miles to the Sam McDonald County Park entrance, bearing right at the sharp junction with Alpine Road a mile from Highway 84. The park entrance comes up quickly on the right; there is a parking fee. Note that registration at Memorial County Park entrance station (when it's staffed) is required for overnight use of the trail camp—the entrance station is located 3.5 miles past the trailhead on Pescadero Road.

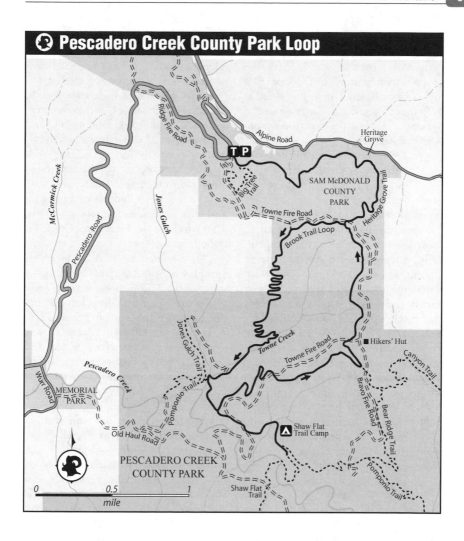

② Pescadero Creek County Park Loop

Hiking It

To travel on single-track trails rather than fire roads, the hike begins on a more circuitous route through Heritage Grove rather than following the more direct route along Towne Fire Road. This choice adds 1.6 miles to the total trip distance, but the rewards of an old-growth redwood grove and bonus views into Pescadero Creek canyon merit the effort. To avoid this extra distance, begin on Towne Fire Road and follow it a little less than a mile to the first junction for Brook Trail Loop, located on the right at the beginning of the open fields atop Towne Ridge.

At the trailhead, tall redwoods tower over the large parking lot (0.0/650'), and several common redwood forest constituents can be identified in front of the intermittently staffed ranger station. Two bigleaf maple trees curve overhead, the fuzzy soft leaves of hazel bushes grow in the understory, and cloverlike redwood sorrel coats the ground with a miniature forest two inches high. Broad Towne Fire Road is prominently signed at the head of the parking area, but the described route begins instead on single-track Heritage Grove Trail, found closer to the parking lot entrance by an area trail map.

California bay and canyon live oak grow overhead as the trail immediately drops to Pescadero Road. Cross it and continue through the gate. The large, spiny leaves of tanoak appear immediately, waving beneath several majestic ancient redwoods. Enormous sword ferns and a carpet of redwood sorrel enrich the world with green as the trail reaches the junction with Big Tree Trail (0.1/620'). Bear left. Contouring slowly uphill through thick forest, the trail next reaches Heritage Grove and a posted junction (1.4/670')—bear right toward the Hikers' Hut. You may want to drop your pack for a moment before continuing, however, and turn left to stroll the short distance to the main flat of Heritage Grove, a 37-acre old-growth stand protected through the efforts of a local citizens' group.

Back on the main route, the trail steadily climbs, offering a few fleeting glimpses north across Alpine Creek drainage, and then encounters a gate immediately before reaching the ridgetop and intersection with Towne Fire Road (1.9/1,150'). The Hikers' Hut awaits here (visit **www. lomaprieta.sierraclub.org** or call (650) 390-8411, ext. 393 for more information). Next cross Towne Fire Road to find the junction with Brook Trail Loop, and turn right (the return route is to the left), passing along the edge

of open meadows regularly rooted by nonnative wild pigs. The trail parallels telephone poles and the fire road as it winds along a mixed-evergreen environment populated by coyote brush, blackberry brambles, bracken fern, madrone, ceanothus, Douglas-fir, and moss-festooned coast live oak. Excellent views south into Pescadero Creek canyon open up along this section— the region of Portola Redwoods State Park is visible a few miles upstream and lofty Butano Ridge rises more than 1,500 feet above Pescadero Creek on the opposite slopes.

After reentering a shady forest of Douglas-fir, the trail reaches another junction (2.3/1,060') connecting back to Towne Fire Road. Bear left and begin the steep descent on Brook Trail. A long series of switchbacks slowly drops into an ever-wetter world and suddenly the mixed-evergreen forest of Douglas-fir becomes dominated by redwood trees (3.5/700'), their draping shields of foliage coloring the forest a vibrant green. As the trail steadily descends into the Towne Creek drainage, watch for some old-growth redwoods—several approach eight feet in diameter. Crossing the creek gully on a small bridge, the trail briefly parallels the watercourse and then hits a road junction (4.5/300'). Turn right here and then take the immediate left on the spur trail posted for Brook Trail Loop to cross above the deep gully of Jones Gulch and reach the intersection with Pomponio Trail (4.6/280'). Head left (downstream) to cross above a magical waterfall grotto on another Towne Creek Bridge.

Continue on Pomponio Trail as it climbs beneath some impressive redwoods and crosses a well-marked fire road until the trail reaches the second junction with Brook Trail Loop (4.8/400')—your return trail. To reach the trail camp from here, follow the numerous signs for Pomponio Trail as it closely parallels and then briefly follows an adjacent fire road before reaching a posted short spur trail to the camp area (5.4/400'). Shaw Flat Trail descends a short quarter mile past camp to Pescadero Creek and provides the easiest access to creek water.

After a revitalizing night, return to the closer Brook Trail Loop Junction (6.0/400'), and bear right (uphill) to begin the climb back out. As you slowly ascend, so goes the transition from lush redwood forest—and some nice ancient groves—to a mixed-evergreen forest of massive Douglas-firs and moss-encrusted, Hydralike bay trees. The trail crosses Towne Fire Road once as it ascends (6.8/780') to reach the junction with Bear Ridge Trail (7.5/1,020'). Turn left to remain on Brook Trail Loop as it crosses Towne

Fire Road again and contours north just below the ridgeline. The slopes are steep around an enchanting redwood grove, and a picnic site offers vistas south as the trail winds among a much drier chaparral community of coffee berry, coyote brush, bracken fern, and sticky monkeyflower to rejoin the earlier junction with Heritage Grove Trail (8.6/1,150'). From here, return either via Towne Fire Road to reach the parking lot in 1.2 miles (9.8/650'), bearing right at the Horse Camp along the way; or along earlier Heritage Grove Trail to end your journey (10.5/650').

Giving Back

San Mateo County Parks Foundation provides financial support for the recreational, environmental, and educational programs and projects of the San Mateo County Parks and Recreation Department. Contact them or learn more at 215 Bay Road, Menlo Park, CA 94025; (650) 321-5812; or **www. supportparks.org.**

13 Portola Redwoods State Park

RATINGS	Scenery **5** Difficulty **3** Solitude **4**
ROUND-TRIP DISTANCE	5.0 miles to trail camp; 12.0 miles to Peters Creek Grove
ELEVATION GAIN/LOSS	+650'/–650' to trail camp; +2,250'/–2,250' to grove
RECOMMENDED MAP	*Portola Redwoods State Park Map* by California State Parks and the Portola and Castle Rock Foundation
BEST TIMES	May through November
AGENCY	Portola Redwoods State Park, (650) 948-9098, **www.parks.ca.gov.** Visitor center is open daily in summer; in the off-season it's open Friday–Sunday and sporadically the rest of week.
PERMIT	Reservations are required for Slate Creek Trail Camp and can be made up to two months in advance by calling (831) 338-8861, Monday–Friday 10 a.m.–5 p.m. Trail camp is closed November through April.

Highlights

The cloak of the redwood forest hushes sound, diffuses light, and radiates life. Travel through a dense canopy of regeneration to a shady trail camp, your base for exploring a distant stand of huge old-growth redwoods: the lightly traveled Peters Creek Grove.

Hike Overview

The journey to Slate Creek Trail Camp winds through a thick redwood forest rejuvenating from recent logging activity. From camp, a moderately strenuous 7-mile round-trip to Peters Creek Grove rewards with ancient majesty. Nearby Slate Creek is delightful as well and makes for good adventuring closer to camp. Expect damp, cool conditions year-round as the forest canopy blocks out most sun and is often infused with fog or rain.

Trail Camp

Slate Creek Trail Camp features six sites spread along a broad forested saddle and populated with a thick forest of young redwood, Douglas-fir, and tanoak. Water is *not* available in camp, but perennial Slate Creek can be accessed a third of a mile and a hundred feet down from camp on Slate Creek Trail. Picnic tables and an outhouse are provided, but there are no food lockers to protect your victuals—*hang your food or it may be gone in the morning.* The trail camp receives moderate use, mostly on summer weekends. Except for the busiest summer weekends and holidays, however, it is seldom full. *Campfires and dogs are prohibited.*

Sites cost $15 per night (maximum six people per site). You must mail an $8 nonrefundable reservation fee to secure the site (21600 Big Basin Way, Boulder Creek, CA 95006). Pay your camping fees at the visitor center once you arrive.

Getting There

Take Highway 35 to the turnoff for Alpine Road, located 6 miles north of the junction of Highways 35 and 9 and 7 miles south of the junction of Highways 35 and 84. Head south on Alpine Road, and in 2.5 miles bear left on Price Avenue to continue downward for another 3 miles to the visitor center. Note that the access road is steep and winding, and *RVs and trailers are not recommended.* Backpackers must register at the visitor center before proceeding to the trailhead, on the left just past the campground entrance and posted for Slate Creek Trail.

Hiking It

The trail begins on Slate Creek Trail (0.0/430'), passing redwoods, canyon live oak, and the ubiquitous spiny leaves of small tanoak trees and shrubs. You quickly reach the junction with Old Tree Trail, which continues straight on a short and worthwhile side trip. Bear left toward Slate Creek Trail Camp. The single-track trail immediately climbs past Douglas-firs and continues uphill past a spur trail from the campground on the left (0.5/670'). You next pass a pleasant bench in Bolton Memorial Grove before several quick switchbacks lead to a more level traverse punctuated by the appearance of California bay. Continue on Slate Creek Trail as Summit Trail joins from the right (1.3/930'), an alternate route back to the park road for the return trip. From here it's a long traverse atop often steep slopes to Slate Creek Trail Camp (2.5/1,000') and the junction for Peters Creek on Bear Creek Trail. Slate Creek can be accessed a short distance farther on Slate Creek Trail at a former mill site.

⊙ Portola Redwoods State Park

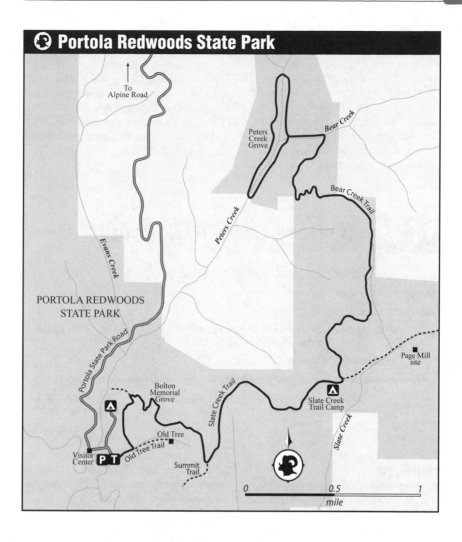

To
Alpine Road

Peters
Creek
Grove

Bear Creek

Peters Creek

Bear Creek Trail

Evans Creek

PORTOLA REDWOODS
STATE PARK

Portola State Park Road

Page Mill
site

Bolton
Memorial
Grove

Slate Creek Trail

Slate Creek
Trail Camp

Old Tree

Old Tree Trail

Slate Creek

Visitor
Center **P** **T**

Summit
Trail

0   0.5   1

mile

To continue to Peters Creek Grove, bravely pass the CAUTION sign on Bear Creek Trail and begin the STRENOUS 7-MILE ROUND-TRIP HIKE FROM THIS POINT. Winding along Bear Creek, you may notice the decaying automobile among the bigleaf maple and hazel by the creek before breaking out into an opening thick with poison oak. A huge, moss-draped coast live oak is on the right past this clearing near the high point of the hike (1,450') before the trail passes through thick Douglas-fir and begins the descent into the Peters Creek drainage. A brief view of the valley appears along the ridge beyond a few California buckeye, but the steady drop is mostly uneventful . . . until the redwoods reappear.

From the junction at the bottom for the Peters Creek Loop (5.0/740') either direction is good but going left first saves the fattest trees in Peters Creek Grove for the very end. The loop twice crosses Peters Creek; you may have to ford it following winter storms. The enormous specimens upstream approach 10 feet in diameter and exhibit striking similarity to their even larger cousins, the giant sequoia. They owe their size to the ideal growing conditions and constant water supply.

Giving Back

Portola and Castle Rock Foundation supports interpretive projects at Portola Redwoods and Castle Rock state parks and publishes maps, brochures, and interpretive materials for the parks. Contact them or learn more at (650) 948-9098 or **www.parks.ca.gov/default. asp?page_id=22075**.

14 Castle Rock State Park Loop

RATINGS	Scenery **8** Difficulty **5** Solitude **5**
ROUND-TRIP DISTANCE	5.2 miles
ELEVATION GAIN/LOSS	+1,200'/–1,200'
OPTIONAL MAP	*Castle Rock State Park Map* by California State Parks and the Portola and Castle Rock Foundation
BEST TIMES	Year-round
AGENCY	Castle Rock State Park, (408) 867-2952, **www.parks.ca.gov**
PERMIT	Trail campsites are always available on a first-come, first-served basis. Register and pay your overnight fees at the park entrance station.

Highlights

A short backpacking trip to a lightly traveled trail camp, this adventure rewards with fantastic sandstone boulders and towering views of the San Lorenzo River and Pescadero Creek watersheds.

Hike Overview

The hike traverses the upper tier of the Santa Cruz Mountains, running high along the western slopes to reach a pleasantly secluded trail camp. Summer fog can obscure the hike's incredible views and winter storms can be heavy, but there is no bad time to visit. Crowds on the trail are relatively light,

though the rock formations close to the park entrance attract climbers and scramblers on the weekends.

Trail Camps

Castle Rock Trail Camp offers 20 sites spread between two areas—**Main Camp** and **Frog Flat Camp**—at an elevation of 2,400 feet in thick knobcone pines, madrone, live oaks, and chaparral. It is the only trail camp in the Bay Area that occasionally permits campfires— firewood is even available for purchase right at the trail camp. *(Campfires are prohibited during wildfire season, typically June through November; call ahead for current information.)* Piped drinking

⊙ Castle Rock State Park Loop

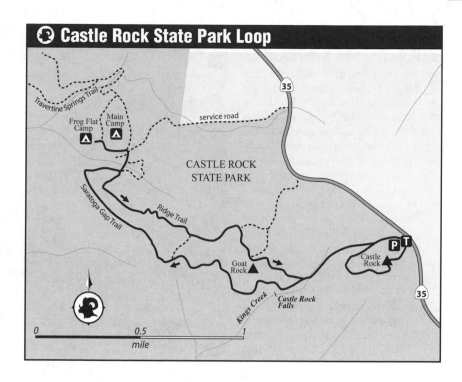

water is available at the trail camp, as is a large sleeping shelter for use during inclement weather. Sites cost $15 per night and include trailhead parking for one vehicle (extra vehicles cost $8 each); register at the park entrance station upon arrival. A maximum of six people are allowed per site.

Getting There
Take Highway 35 south of the Highway 9 junction for 2.5 miles. The posted entrance and parking area are located on the west side of the road.

Hiking It
A small forest of signs marks the trailhead at the edge of the parking lot (0.0/3,070'). While the direct route to the trail camp proceeds straight on Saratoga Gap Trail, the park's fasci-

nating sandstone formations are accessed via a short half-mile loop that rejoins the main trail a short distance ahead. It is an attraction well worth visiting—those arriving late in the day should consider exploring this area on the return trip.

To begin among the boulders, bear left at the trailhead toward Castle Rock, turn right on the immediate fire road, and quickly reach the first wild stone pile on the left. From here interlaced paths wind past a variety of outcrops before reaching Castle Rock itself, an apartment-sized monolith deeply gouged by erosion. After exploring this unusual geologic world, proceed the short distance to Saratoga Gap Trail and bear left.

To head directly to the campground from the trailhead (0.0/3,070'), proceed straight on Saratoga Gap Trail as it passes through a mixed-evergreen forest dominated by the drooping evergreen branches of Douglas-fir, the large spiny leaves of tanoak, and the twisting trunks of madrone. A trailside understory of blackberry and poison oak discourages a departure from the soft path as it begins its descent into the Kings Creek drainage, one of the uppermost headwaters of the San Lorenzo River.

Dropping into a dry gully, the trail quickly passes a junction on the left for Castle Rock (0.1/3,000') where those exploring the sandstone formations rejoin the main trail. The trail continues downward and a spring soon appears, feeding Kings Creek. The broad leaves of bigleaf maple appear overhead and thick clumps of sword ferns sprout along the moist creek bed. Crossing the creek, the trail reaches the junction with Ridge Trail (0.5/2,730') and the beginning of the loop. The hike can easily be completed in either direction; this description continues on Saratoga Gap Trail and returns via Ridge Trail.

A few young redwoods join large Douglas-firs as Saratoga Gap Trail continues briefly along the creek to reach the sheer overlook for the thin cascade of Castle Rock Falls (0.7/2,700'). From here Kings Creek plummets downward and drops more than a thousand vertical feet in less than a mile. Heading away from the creek, Saratoga Gap Trail quickly passes onto drier slopes where coffee berry, toyon, and fragrant California bay appear—plants better adapted to a world of less moisture.

The hike traverses steep slopes, passing through a world of chaparral protruded by sandstone boulders, and enters a stand of rustling black oaks shortly before reaching a connector trail on the right leading to nearby

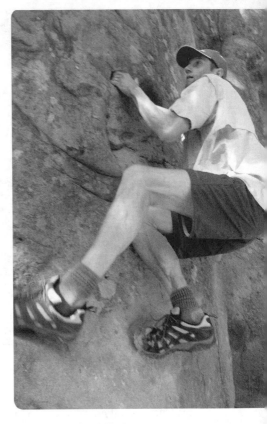

Bouldering on Castle Rock

Ridge Trail (1.5/2,560'). Continue straight on Saratoga Gap Trail as spectacular views soon open into the heart of the Santa Cruz Mountains.

Looking south beyond the vast drainage of the San Lorenzo River, the Monterey peninsula can be identified across Monterey Bay on clear days (a distance of more than 40 miles). To the west, the low ridge separating the San Lorenzo River and Pescadero Creek watersheds is apparent; the Skyline-to-the-Sea Trail (see page 116) follows this divide en route to Big Basin Redwoods State Park. Tall Bonny Doon Ridge hems the San Lorenzo River to the southwest, while Butano Ridge rises above Pescadero Creek to the west. The deep canyon of Pescadero Creek curves out-of-sight to the northwest, harboring many an overnight outdoor adventure in its recesses—Portola Redwoods State Park, Memorial County Park, and Pescadero Creek County Park all await exploration.

Now gradually descending, you pass through chaparral thick with coyote brush and poison oak. Narrow and rocky in places, the trail winds along sheer slopes before turning sharply right to pass through a suddenly thick forest of tanoak and madrone before reaching the junction with Ridge Trail (2.5/2,400'). To reach the trail camp, bear left, and then left again on the

wide fire road to reach the main area (2.7/2,400'). Knobcone pines abruptly appear beside young Douglas-firs in this section, their twisted architecture and namesake cones making them easy to identify. The 15 sites of the Main Camp area are located nearby off Saratoga Gap Trail, while the five sites of more-removed Frog Flat Camp are located a quarter mile downhill on Service Road Trail, just below the intersection with Frog Flat Trail.

To head home, return to the earlier junction with Ridge Trail (2.9/2,400') and follow Ridge Trail as it climbs briefly through thick forest before emerging at another incredible viewpoint of the Santa Cruz Mountains. Continue on Ridge Trail as it returns

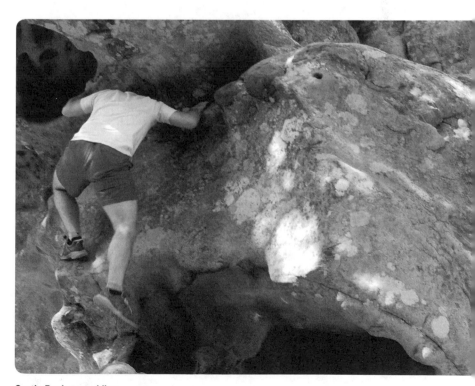

Castle Rock scrambling

THE WILD GEOLOGY OF CASTLE ROCK

Castle Rock State Park perches on the tallest ridgeline in the Santa Cruz Mountains and harbors a geologic wonderland. Heavy winter precipitation (45 to 50 inches annually) falls upon the area's unusually hard sandstone outcrops, creating conditions ideal for some bizarre chemical weathering known as tafoni. As all this rain falls upon the rocks, water seeps inside and dissolves the thin matrix of calcium carbonate that binds the individual sand grains together.

When dry conditions return, the moisture trapped inside the rocks is drawn back to the surface. Its evaporation leaves behind the calcium carbonate as a hard and intricate surface residue. Without the calcium carbonate "glue" to hold them together, the interior sand grains waste away to leave small cavities behind. Over time these cavities can become intricate catacombs, their puckered walls a fascinating honeycomb of pitted rock.

to the forest, climbs along the north side of the ridge, and then reaches the opposite end of the connector trail to Saratoga Gap Trail (3.7/2,700'). Remain on Ridge Trail as it climbs over a black oak-studded knoll to reach a fork (4.0/2,900'). Turn left for a short side-loop that rejoins Ridge Trail in 0.3 mile after passing an informative interpretive shelter. Ridge Trail continues to the right, passing the return trail from the interpretive shelter (4.2/2,960'), and then reaches the junction to exciting Goat Rock (4.3/2,920'). Another climbing destination, the rounded pinnacle of Goat Rock and its surrounding viewpoints can be accessed via numerous use trails and thrilling rock scrambles. After enjoying the most intense verticality of the trip, continue on Ridge Trail as it slowly descends along a narrow, rocky route to rejoin Saratoga Gap Trail (4.4/2,730') and the final climb back to the parking lot (5.2/3,070').

Giving Back

Portola and Castle Rock Foundation supports interpretive projects at Portola Redwoods and Castle Rock state parks and publishes maps, brochures, and interpretive materials for the parks. Contact the foundation or learn more at (650) 948-9098 or **www.parks.ca.gov/ default.asp?page_id=22075**.

Sempervirens Fund is dedicated to preserving, expanding, and linking parklands in the Santa Cruz Mountains. Contact them or learn more at (650) 949-1453 or **www.sempervirens.org**.

15 Big Basin Redwoods State Park:
BASIN TRAIL LOOP

RATINGS	Scenery **7** Difficulty **5** Solitude **7**
ROUND-TRIP DISTANCE	11.6 miles
ELEVATION GAIN/LOSS	+1,500'/−1,500'
RECOMMENDED MAP	*Castle Rock State Park Map* and *Big Basin Redwoods State Park Map* by California State Parks and *Trail Map of the Santa Cruz Mountains 2* by the Sempervirens Fund
BEST TIMES	May through October
AGENCY	Big Basin Redwoods State Park, (831) 338-8860, **www.bigbasin.org**, **www.parks.ca.gov**
PERMIT	Reservations are required for Lane Trail Camp and can be made up to two months in advance by calling (831) 338-8861, Monday–Friday 10 a.m.–5 p.m. Lane Trail Camp is closed November through April.

Highlights

The northeast section of Big Basin harbors spectacular old-growth, gurgling streams, and a remote trail camp far removed from the bustle that permeates much of the park.

Hike Overview

This hike provides an excellent—and much less-traveled—alternative to the popular Sunset Camp loop, yet still offers the full range of Big Basin highlights. It begins from Big Basin headquarters and heads east alongside the tranquil waters and eye-popping old-growth of Opal Creek. After 2.5 miles of forest primeval, the journey embarks on a 6-mile loop around the northeast corner of the park to Lane Camp, the park's most isolated trail camp, then returns along Opal Creek.

Trail Camp

Lane Trail Camp offers six sites in a dense forest of tanoak with small live oaks, madrone, Douglas-fir, and redwoods interspersed. Quiet and solitude

are usually in abundance, but water is *not*. A few ephemeral trickles can be found during rainy season, but bring all the water you will need; the last reliable spot to fill up is Opal Creek. *Dogs and campfires are prohibited.*

Sites cost $15 per night (maximum six people per site). You must mail an $8 nonrefundable reservation fee to secure the site (21600 Big Basin Way, Boulder Creek, CA 95006). Pay your camping fees at Big Basin headquarters once you arrive. For more information, visit **www.bigbasin.org**.

Note that Jay Trail Camp near park headquarters may only be used by "en route" backpackers on the Skyline-to-the-Sea Trail (see page 116); for a late day arrival, consider staying at one of the park's drive-in campgrounds (reservations essential, 800-444-7275, **www.reserveamerica.com**).

Getting There

Take Highway 236 west from one of two junctions on Highway 9. Approaching from Highway 35 to the

⚙ Big Basin Redwoods State Park: Basin Trail Loop

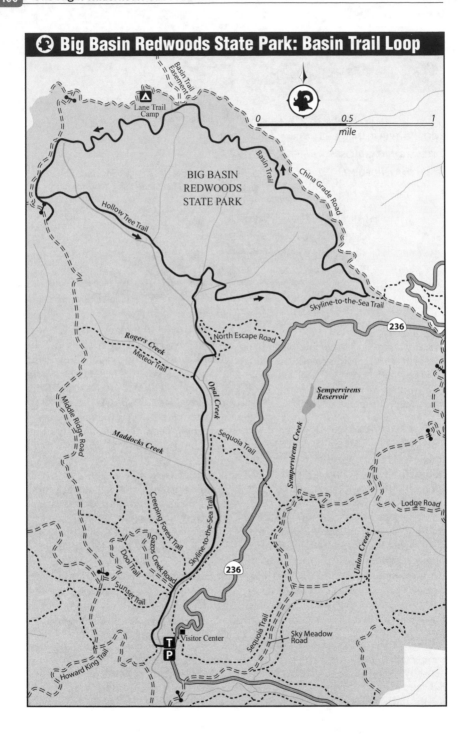

north, the upper turnoff is 5.8 miles below the junction of Highways 35 and 9. From this turnoff, Highway 236 is a one-lane twister that reaches the visitor center in 8.0 miles—*RVs and trailers are not recommended.* Approaching from the south, the lower turnoff is in Boulder Creek. This easier driving section of Highway 236 reaches park headquarters in 9.0 miles. The trailhead is across the road from the visitor center. Water is readily available. Public transportation is available to the park from downtown Santa Cruz on weekends with the Santa Cruz Metro bus service (**www.scmtd.com**).

Hiking It

From the trailhead parking lot across from the visitor center, take broad Redwood Trail beyond the restrooms, and cross Opal Creek to meet the Skyline-to-the-Sea Trail (0.1/950'). Bear right on the easy-cruising level path, soon passing three closely spaced junctions on the left: Dool Trail (0.4/960'), named for the third park warden of Big Basin Redwoods State Park; Gazos Creek Road (0.5/970'); and then Creeping Forest Trail (0.6/960').

Look for the soft leaves of hazel bushes as you continue on the often muddy trail, cruising close to Opal Creek and past the fluted trunks of giant redwoods. You next reach Maddocks Creek, where an interpretive placard tells the story of an early settler who built an entire cabin from a single redwood tree. Soon you encounter the park road again at a bridge crossing (1.4/1,040'), where you remain on the left (west) side of Opal Creek to follow the Skyline-to-the-Sea Trail.

The route next passes Meteor Trail on the left (1.7/1,070'), momentarily joins the road, then briefly parallels the road to reach a paved bridge over Opal Creek. Bear left to cross the bridge. You next reach paved North Escape Road near an informative kiosk (1.9/1,060') and then follow the burbling stream past large chain ferns and humongous redwoods. Cross Opal Creek once again on a wooden walkway.

The route next encounters the junction for Hollow Tree Trail on the left (2.4/1,270'), your return route. Remain for now on the Skyline-to-the-Sea Trail as it quickly crosses two small headwater trickles of Opal Creek, turns uphill, and curves left to leave the lush redwood forest. Bid farewell for now to the magnificent old-growth forest as you climb into a new ecosystem.

Say hello instead to dense chaparral punctuated by spindly knobcone pines. As you traverse the slopes, views appear for the first time over the rolling forests. You then reach the junction with the Basin Trail (4.2/1,980'), where you turn left to head toward Lane Trail Camp.

Basin Trail begins an undulating, gradually rising traverse along the uppermost slopes of the Waddell Creek watershed. After passing several of the many excellent viewpoints found along this section, the trail enters the shade of dense madrone trees and continues through a more diverse mixed-evergreen forest of Douglas-fir, tanoak, coast live oak, and the occasional redwood. Cresting a small rise, the trail then curves right and enters a region marked in recent years by wildfire. After passing the flame-blackened trunks of gnarled redwoods on a north-facing hillside, the trail returns to the south-facing slopes and a drier world dominated by knobcone pines.

A spindly conifer with namesake cones bursting from everywhere (including on branches and trunks), knobcone pines survive through a process called serotiny—their cones open only during wildfire. Freshly opened cones populate the burned-out, nutrient-rich soil with a massive influx of seeds, resulting in a region dominated by young trees. As the trail passes through this unusual forest, chaparral, such as manzanita and sticky monkeyflower, can be found intermixed in the dry environment.

Undulating slowly upward the trail next winds through unusual sandstone outcrops dotted with open chaparral and excellent views. Following this rocky and boulder-strewn section, the trail returns to shady north-facing slopes where redwoods instantly reappear. The trail passes three small ephemeral creeks in a forest of tanoak, madrone, and live oak, and then turns abruptly uphill to follow a narrow creek gully to reach a four-way junction (7.3/2,280'). Hollow Tree Trail—your continuing route—goes left, but Lane Trail Camp is straight ahead, a short 0.1 mile from this junction on a narrow, slightly overgrown trail. A right turn at the junction takes you to China Grade Road and the start of the Basin Trail Easement, connecting Portola Redwoods and Big Basin Redwoods state parks.

Begin the return to headquarters on Hollow Tree Trail as it winds through thick vegetation regenerating from the recent wildfire. Views are generally obscured by the dense underbrush as the trail contours through the burn zone—blackened young redwoods less than a foot in diameter indicate how recently the area charred. A few old-growth redwood survivors appear intermittently as well, demonstrating their resiliency and resistance to wildfire with burn marks

more than 30 feet off the ground. The trail's final view, looking down the drainage of Opal Creek and the direction of descent, soon opens up. After crossing the Opal Creek headwaters by a massive redwood tree, the trail ends its contouring traverse by the large metal detritus of Johansen Shingle Mill (built in 1927). Massive boilers and large metal pieces can be explored just off the trail near a memorial bench that asks, EVERYBODY HAPPY?

Passing beneath young redwood forest, the trail then drops steeply down the narrow creek gully and quickly reaches a short connector trail leading to Middle Ridge Fire Road (8.8/1,780'). Bearing left, the trail continues its steep descent, makes two creek crossings, and then parallels the flowing stream as it babbles among moss-coated boulders. Crossing yet another small tributary, the trail contours through a lush, less-burned forest before rejoining the Skyline-to-the Sea Trail (9.2/1,270'). Bear right and retrace your steps to the trailhead (11.6/950').

Giving Back

Mountain Parks Foundation provides resources that expands visitors' knowledge and appreciation of the natural environment and cultural heritage of Henry Cowell and Big Basin Redwoods state parks. Contact them or learn more at (831) 535-3174 or **www. mountainparks.org**.

Sempervirens Fund is dedicated to preserving, expanding, and linking parklands in the Santa Cruz Mountains. Contact them or learn more at (650) 949-1453 or **www.sempervirens.org**.

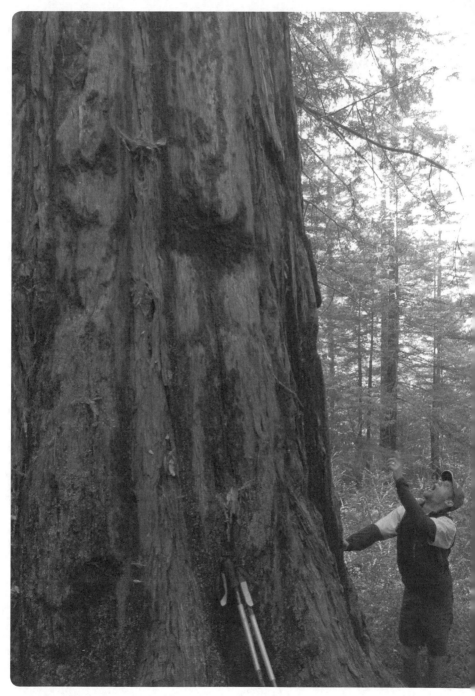

That's a big tree!

16 Big Basin Redwoods State Park:
SUNSET TRAIL CAMP LOOP

RATINGS	Scenery **10** Difficulty **6** Solitude **1**
ROUND-TRIP DISTANCE	10.0 miles
ELEVATION GAIN/LOSS	+3,300'/–3,300'
OPTIONAL MAPS	*Big Basin Redwoods State Park Map* by California State Parks and *Trail Map of the Santa Cruz Mountains 2* by the Sempervirens Fund
BEST TIMES	May through October
AGENCY	Big Basin Redwoods State Park, (831) 338-8860, **www.bigbasin.org, www.parks.ca.gov**
PERMIT	Reservations are required for Sunset Trail Camp and can be made up to two months in advance by calling (831) 338-8861, Monday–Friday 10 a.m.–5 p.m. The trail camp is closed November through April.

Highlights

A continuous forest primeval, Big Basin Redwoods State Park is a green blaze of life. Yes, the park is popular and the waterfalls are a common destination. And yes, it's worth it.

Hike Overview

The hike loops through towering old-growth redwood forest and past three waterfalls—Silver Falls, Golden Falls, and photogenic Berry Creek Falls—reaching Sunset Trail Camp near the journey's midpoint. No matter what day you come, other people will be on the trail. Weekend crowds can be especially thick.

Trail Camp

Sunset Trail Camp is situated in a pleasant, second-growth redwood forest and offers 10 sites spread between two areas. Sunset is the park's most popular trail camp because of its location near the waterfalls, its access via beautiful old-growth redwood forest, and its ideal location for overnight loop trips

from Big Basin headquarters. It is often full—reserve well in advance. Water is *not* available in camp, but perennial Berry Creek is only a third of a mile away. *Pets and campfires are prohibited.*

Sites cost $15 per night (maximum six people per site). You must mail an $8 nonrefundable reservation fee to secure the site (21600 Big Basin Way, Boulder Creek, CA 95006). Pay your camping fees at Big Basin headquarters once you arrive. For more information, visit **www.bigbasin.org**.

Note that Jay Trail Camp near park headquarters may only be used by "en route" backpackers on the Skyline-to-the-Sea Trail (see page 116); for a late day arrival, consider staying at one of the park's drive-in campgrounds (reservations essential, 800-444-7275, **www.reserveamerica.com**).

Getting There

Take Highway 236 west from one of two junctions on Highway 9. Approaching from Highway 35 to the north, the upper turnoff is 5.8 miles

⚙ Big Basin Redwoods State Park: Sunset Trail Camp Loop

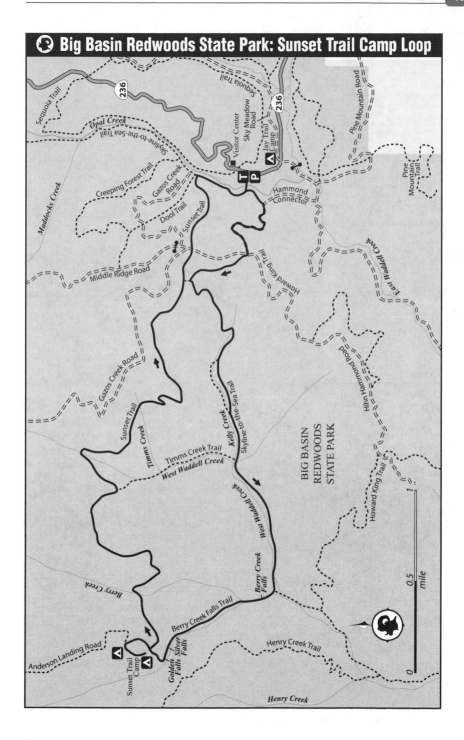

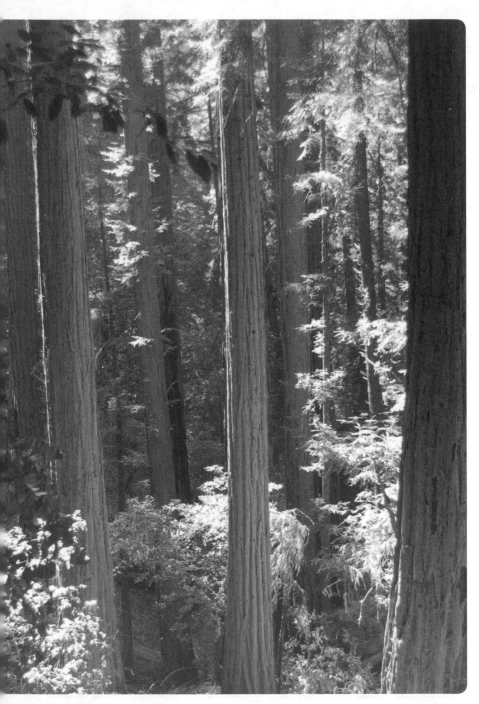

Sun-dappled redwood grove

A MIGHTY STAND

Established in 1902, Big Basin was the first state park created to protect old-growth redwood forest in the Santa Cruz Mountains. In fact, the 3,800 acres initially set aside as parkland were the very first to protect coast redwoods anywhere! The park holdings have since expanded, and the total park area now exceeds 19,000 acres, stretching from the Pacific Ocean at the mouth of Waddell Creek to the heart of the Santa Cruz Mountains. The old-growth redwood forest is extensive and unmatched in total area for hundreds of miles up the coast.

below the junction of Highways 35 and 9. From this turnoff, Highway 236 is a one-lane twister that reaches the visitor center in 8.0 miles—*RVs and trailers are not recommended.* Approaching from the south, the lower turnoff is in Boulder Creek. This easier driving section of Highway 236 reaches the visitor center and headquarters complex in 9.0 miles. The trailhead is across the road from the visitor center. Water is readily available. Public transportation is available to the park from downtown Santa Cruz on weekends with the Santa Cruz Metro bus service (**www.scmtd.com**).

Hiking It

From the trailhead (0.0/990'), take broad Redwood Trail beyond the restrooms and across Opal Creek to your junction with the Skyline-to-the-Sea Trail. Your return trail joins from the right, but you head left, passing some large Douglas-firs and many tanoaks whose toothed leaves wave everywhere. Continue toward Berry Creek Falls at the next junction with Hammond Connector (0.1/970'), and begin a steady climb out of the East Waddell Creek drainage. After several switchbacks, the trail crests into the West Waddell Creek drainage at a junction with Howard King Trail

(0.8/1,320'). A sign warns of the strenuous hiking ahead.

Continuing straight, you immediately descend and soon pass a connector to Sunset Trail on the right (1.2/1,170'). The trail winds downward though a spectacular old-growth forest dominated by the thick trunks of mature redwoods—dozens of perfect trees fill the forest view in every direction. After crossing a bridge over Kelly Creek (note the profusion of giant chain ferns in the creek bed), the trail then begins a traverse above the waterway. An alternate route soon splits right to more closely follow the stream's course before rejoining the main trail 0.4 mile later.

At the next junction (2.5/530'), Timms Creek Trail makes a hair-raising stream crossing on slippery logs before heading upward along upper West Waddell Creek to connect with Sunset Trail. The canyon gets narrower and rockier as you continue downstream on the Skyline-to-the-Sea Trail, drop to cross West Waddell Creek, briefly climb to reach a tantalizing view of Berry Creek Falls, and then descend to reach the junction with Berry Creek Falls Trail (3.9/350') at the confluence of the two creeks. Turn right toward the falls, leaving the Skyline-to-the-Sea

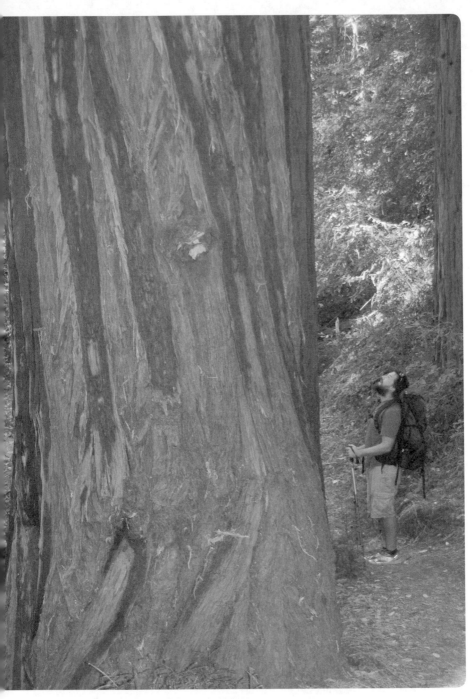

An old-growth redwood dwarfs a passing hiker.

Trail to its journey toward the ocean, here less than 6 miles away.

From the creek confluence, Berry Creek Falls Trail immediately leads to a large wooden viewing platform for the waterfall. Unless a recent winter storm has swollen the waters, Berry Creek Falls are thin and drop in small cascades that mist the surrounding greenery. Thimbleberry and sword fern coat the damp ground below; tanoak and redwoods rise above; and five-finger ferns wave from the surrounding steep, mossy slopes.

Passing near the bottom of the waterfall, the trail then climbs left above the falls, and crosses Berry Creek. The muddy track stays close to the water and soon reaches Silver Falls, a small cascade falling over exposed sedimentary rock representative of the Santa Cruz Mountains geology.

The bedrock of the Santa Cruz Mountains is granite formed some 100 million years ago near the location of today's southern Sierra Nevada. When the San Andreas Fault became active, this piece of land began moving slowly northwest, becoming submerged beneath the sea as it went. Sand and mud settled from the ocean on this underwater surface, forming thick layers of loosely consolidated sandstone and mudstone. Within the past 4 million years, a change in the geometry of the San Andreas Fault thrust these layers aboveground, folding them into the Santa Cruz Mountains and exposing the muddy layers to your boots.

After climbing above Silver Falls on a thrilling section protected with cables, the trail then reaches Golden Falls, which pours in waterslide fashion over brilliant orange sandstone. The trail next curves right to climb out of the narrow creek canyon and reach the junction with Sunset Trail (4.9/770').

To reach Sunset Trail Camp, bear left and follow the narrow trail as it climbs up steep slopes through a suddenly drier world of knobcone pines, manzanita, live oak, and golden chinquapin to reach Anderson Landing Road in 0.2 mile by a fragrant outhouse (5.1/1,010'). Six sites are available directly across the road (follow the signs), while the remaining four are located 0.1 mile and 70 feet lower, surrounding the large turnout and end of Anderson Landing Road.

To return to Big Basin headquarters, return to Sunset Trail (5.3/770') and follow it east, crossing Berry Creek on a solid wooden bridge before weaving over a small divide separating West Waddell and Berry creeks. Fleeting views of both drainages open up before the trail descends to the Timms Creek Trail junction (6.8/780'). A long, undulating, and rising traverse from here along Sunset Trail passes the earlier connector trail (9.0/1,200'), then Middle Ridge Road (9.2/1,340'), and finally hits Dool Trail immediately before returning to the Skyline-to-the-Sea Trail (9.7/960'). Turn right and proceed 0.3 mile to reach the earlier junction for Redwood Trail and Big Basin headquarters (10.0/990').

Giving Back

Mountain Parks Foundation provides resources that expand visitors' knowledge and appreciation of the natural environment and cultural heritage of Henry Cowell and Big Basin Redwoods state parks. Contact the foundation or learn more at (831) 535-3174 or **www.mountainparks.org**.

Sempervirens Fund is dedicated to preserving, expanding, and linking parklands in the Santa Cruz Mountains. Contact the group or learn more about them at (650) 949-1453 or **www.sempervirens.org**.

17   Big Basin Redwoods State Park:
INLAND FROM THE SEA

RATINGS	Scenery **7** Difficulty **4** Solitude **4**
ROUND-TRIP DISTANCES	2.0 miles to Alder Trail Camp
	2.4 miles to Twin Redwoods Trail Camp
	11.6 miles to Berry Creek Falls
	14.0 miles to Sunset Trail Camp
ELEVATION GAIN/LOSS	+170'/–170' to Alder Trail Camp
	+200'/–200' to Twin Redwoods Trail Camp
	+500'/–500' to Berry Creek Falls
	+1,150'/–1,150' to Sunset Trail Camp
OPTIONAL MAPS	*Big Basin Redwoods State Park Map* by California State Parks and *Trail Map of the Santa Cruz Mountains 2* by the Sempervirens Fund
BEST TIMES	May through October
AGENCY	Big Basin Redwoods State Park, (831) 338-8860, **www.bigbasin.org**, **www.parks.ca.gov**
PERMIT	Reservations are required for trail camps and can be made up to two months in advance by calling (831) 338-8861, Monday–Friday 10 a.m.–5 p.m. Trail camps are closed November through April.

Highlights
Waddell Creek emerges from old-growth redwood forest, flows through the broad valley of Rancho del Oso, and ends its journey at Waddell Beach. The Skyline-to-the-Sea Trail winds alongside and provides coastside access to the magnificent waterfalls and old-growth forests of central Big Basin Redwoods State Park. You enjoy rich human history and great ecologic diversity along the way.

Hike Overview
The journey inland passes lightly used Alder and Twin Redwoods trail camps en route to superlative old-growth redwood forest, Berry Creek Falls, and Sunset Trail Camp. For most of its length, the hike follows wide, old ranch roads with minimal elevation gain. The trail is open to bikes for most of its length, though the final half mile to Berry Creek Falls is for hikers only—a rack is provided to store bikes while exploring this section on foot.

The lesser-traveled Rancho del Oso region provides a delightful contrast to the far busier world found inland around the central Big Basin complex on Highway 236. Close to the coast, conditions are typically cool year-round, and fog is common throughout summer. Water is available near the trailhead at Horse Camp. *Fishing is prohibited.*

Trail Camps
Three trail camps are available for overnight use. Two of them—Alder and Twin Redwoods—are located a short hike from the trailhead and provide good options for a late-day start. Sunset Trail Camp is the turnaround point for the hike's out-and-back journey.

Big Basin Redwoods State Park: Inland from the Sea

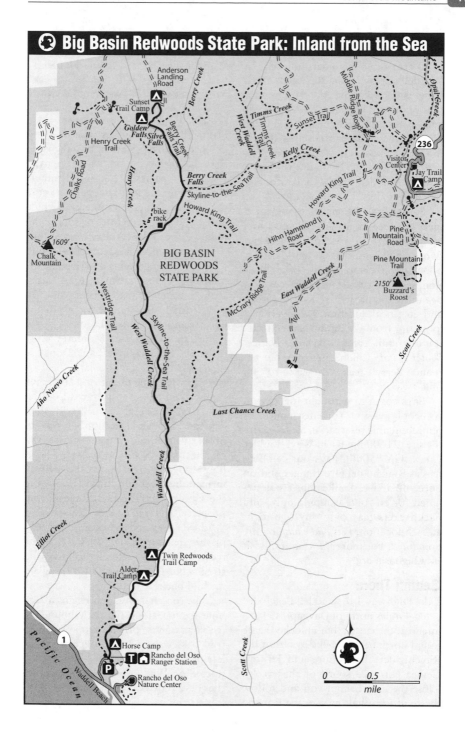

Alder Trail Camp is 1.0 mile from the trailhead and features multiple sites in an area of young alders adjacent to Waddell Creek. **Twin Redwoods Trail Camp** is 0.2 mile past Alder Camp in a shady copse of large bay trees by Waddell Creek. Sites are spacious and offer good privacy. Water is *not* provided at the trail camps, but Waddell Creek is readily accessible. (Treated wastewater flows in Waddell Creek—boil or purify thoroughly).

Sunset Trail Camp is situated in a pleasant, second-growth redwood forest and offers 10 sites spread between two areas. Sunset is the park's most popular trail camp because of its location near the waterfalls, its access via beautiful old-growth redwood forest, and its ideal location for overnight loop trips from Big Basin headquarters. It is often full—reserve well in advance. Water is *not* available in camp, but perennial Berry Creek is only a third of a mile away.

Sites cost $15 per night (maximum six people per site). You must mail an $8 nonrefundable reservation fee to secure the site (21600 Big Basin Way, Boulder Creek, CA 95006). Pay your camping fees at Rancho del Oso Ranger Station once you arrive. Trail camps are designated for en route camping only, and backpackers may only stay one night at each location. *Pets and campfires are prohibited.* For more information, visit **www.bigbasin.org**.

Getting There

Take Highway 1 to Waddell Beach, located 4 miles north of Davenport. Turn inland at the closed (but unlocked) gate found north of Waddell Creek (not the Rancho del Oso Nature and History Center entrance south of the creek). Close the gate behind you and follow the road for a half mile to the Rancho del Oso Ranger Station and parking lot. Public transportation is available to Waddell Beach from downtown Santa Cruz twice daily with the Santa Cruz Metro bus service (**www.scmtd.com**).

Hiking It

From the trailhead by the Rancho del Oso Ranger Station parking area (0.0/20'), begin on the wide, unpaved road as it passes a hikers-only alternate trail on the left. Hikers may enjoy the narrower alternate trail as it winds along the slopes before rejoining the main route near Alder Camp, but the easier—and bike-accessible—route along the broad road is described here.

Horse Camp, a broad, grassy area with a water spigot, appears quickly on the right; the camp is for overnight equestrian use only. Beyond Horse Camp, the trail passes Monterey pine, coast live oak, bay trees, and Douglas-fir as it curves around a large field of coyote brush, wild onion, and abundant lupine. You pass a private road on the right (0.3/40'), climb momentarily, then descend through a section of private property on a right-of-way—please stay on the road. Note the redwood-sided house on your right across the actively farmed fields. Built in 1913, it was the Hoover family's first home on the property. The trail crosses clear-flowing Waddell Creek and passes another gated private road on the right (0.8/30'). Your route now more closely follows the streamcourse, lined with nice Douglas-firs and buckeye trees.

The road narrows and begins a 2.5-mile section along the park boundary (to your right is private property). The trail passes some large concrete pieces left over from a 1930s fish study conducted on Waddell Creek, then enters the first redwood grove of the trip. Here, among healthy second-growth

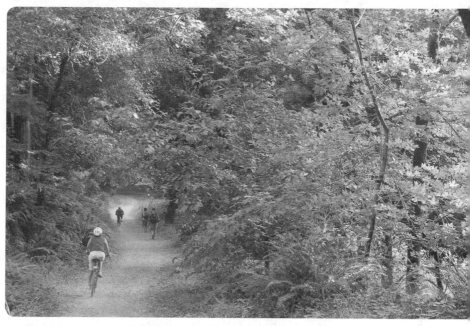

Hikers and bikers share the final section of the Skyline-to-the-Sea Trail.

trees, stands a huge and gnarled redwood known as the Eagle Tree. It is one of the few old-growth trees in this area left uncut by William Waddell's logging operations. Alder Camp is just ahead (1.0/40').

Beyond Alder Camp, you quickly pass the junction for the hikers alternate trail on the left and soon reach Twin Redwoods Camp (1.2/60'). A former Girl Scout summer camp (active from the 1920s through 1957), the location is named for the large, two-headed redwood tree growing nearby.

The trail now leaves private property behind for parkland, soon narrowing to switchbacks over a large 1955 landslide that buried this section of road, some of the most difficult biking of the trip. A short distance later is the site of Camp Herbert (2.5/100'), a former trail camp located just below the out-of-sight confluence of East and West Waddell creeks.

Beyond Camp Herbert, the trail crosses East Waddell Creek on an arched metal bridge and reaches Forks Meadows (2.6/100'). An open area today dotted with coyote brush, Forks Meadow was once the site of three different mills. Waddell constructed the first in 1867 to process the surrounding timber. At the edge of the meadow, McCrary Ridge Trail splits right.

As you continue on the Skyline-to-the-Sea Trail, the surrounding second-growth forest (note how all the trees are the same height) becomes increasingly dense and the canyon begins to palpably narrow. Plant members of the coastal scrub community—blackberry, ceanothus, coffee berry, sticky monkeyflower, stinging nettle, and poison

THE TALE OF WADDELL CREEK

In 1769, Captain Juan Gaspar de Portolá led a Spanish expedition north from Baja California in search of an overland route to Monterey Bay. Mistakenly passing his intended destination, Portolá continued north into the Santa Cruz Mountains. Portolá and his scurvy-ridden men rested for several days in October 1769 at the mouth of Waddell Creek, where the plentiful seafood and small game allowed them to regain their strength. Rejuvenated, the men dubbed the valley Cañada de la Salud ("Canyon of Health"). A few weeks later, they became the first Europeans to discover San Francisco Bay.

Following the gold rush, the easy costal access and giant redwoods attracted William Waddell to the area. Under his direction, the area was heavily logged from 1867 to 1875, and a small town sprang up in the valley to house the forest workers. Waddell was later killed by a grizzly bear. Following this natural retribution, the land was divided into small homesteads populated by hardy folks scrapping a living from the land. Logging continued on a smaller scale until the mid-20th century, and several mills operated along the banks of Waddell Creek.

During the early 1900s, construction of the Ocean Shore Railroad began to connect San Francisco and Santa Cruz. A work camp was established at Waddell Beach in 1904, but the 1906 earthquake disrupted plans and the railroad never made it so far south. The company shut down its limited San Mateo County operations in 1920. Today wind and winter waves occasionally expose remnants of this era near the Waddell Beach parking area.

In 1898, Theodore Hoover first espied the pleasant valley of Waddell Creek and determined to make it his future home. Brother of future president Herbert Hoover, Theodore began acquiring land in 1913 and soon owned roughly 3,000 acres of prime real estate. Stretching from Waddell Beach 5 miles inland along the rich bottomlands and adjacent slopes of Waddell Creek to the boundary with Big Basin Redwoods State Park, it was dubbed Rancho del Oso (or "Ranch of the Bear," despite the fact that the last grizzly in the area was killed during the 1880s). In 1975 the family began transferring ownership of most of the ranch, including the land that connects Big Basin Redwoods State Park to the Pacific Ocean, to California State Parks. The Hoovers still hold parcels of private property and continue to live here as they have for five generations.

Author's note: I adapted this historical information from "Rancho del Oso Trails" by Hulda Hoover McClean, a booklet available, along with more detailed information on the history and hiking trails of the Rancho del Oso area, at the nearby Rancho del Oso Nature and History Center (open noon–4 p.m. weekends). The posted turnoff from Highway 1 is on the south side of Waddell Creek, a short quarter mile from the Waddell Beach parking area.

oak—diminish in the increasingly lush environment.

The trail now parallels West Waddell Creek, winds over several small tributaries, and passes the junction with Henry Creek Trail (5.0/300'). It then crosses the stream on a wooden bridge and reaches a bike rack, which marks the end of the bike-accessible section, as well as the former boundary between Rancho del Oso and Big Basin (5.3/320').

From here the narrower trail descends to recross Waddell Creek, passes the junction with Howard King Trail (5.5/350'), and then crosses the creek one last time on a seasonal bridge; those traveling in the winter months may have to ford the creek. The hike then abruptly transforms into a single-track journey through old-growth redwood forest. The surrounding trees soar with age and grandeur as the trail quickly reaches the junction with Berry Creek Falls Trail by the confluence of West Waddell and Berry creeks (5.7/350').

The Skyline-to-the-Sea Trail continues straight up West Waddell Creek, reaching park headquarters after 4.0 miles of continuous old-growth forest, but you should bear left on Berry Creek Falls Trail to immediately reach the large wooden viewing platform by the falls (5.8/380'). Unless a recent winter storm has swollen the waters, Berry Creek Falls are thin and drop in small cascades that mist the surrounding greenery. Thimbleberry and sword fern coat the damp ground below; tanoak and redwoods rise above; and five-finger ferns wave from the surrounding steep, mossy slopes.

Passing near the bottom of the waterfall, the trail then climbs left above the falls, and crosses Berry Creek. The muddy track stays close to the water and soon reaches Silver Falls, a small cascade falling over exposed sedimentary rock representative of the Santa Cruz Mountain geology.

The bedrock of the Santa Cruz Mountains is granite formed some 100 million years ago near the location of today's southern Sierra Nevada. When the San Andreas Fault became active, this piece of land began moving slowly northwest, becoming submerged beneath the sea as it went. Sand and mud settled from the ocean on this underwater surface, forming thick layers of loosely consolidated sandstone and mudstone. Within the past 4 million years, a change in the geometry of the San Andreas Fault thrust these layers aboveground, folding them into the Santa Cruz Mountains and exposing the muddy layers to your boots.

After climbing above Silver Falls on a thrilling section protected with cables, the trail then reaches Golden Falls, which pours in waterslide fashion over brilliant orange sandstone. The trail next curves right to climb out of the narrow creek canyon and reach the junction with Sunset Trail (6.8/770').

To reach Sunset Trail Camp, bear left and follow the narrow trail as it climbs up steep slopes through a suddenly drier world of knobcone pines, manzanita, live oak, and golden chinquapin to reach Anderson Landing Road in 0.2 mile by a fragrant outhouse (7.0/1,010'). Six sites are available directly across the road (follow the signs), while the remaining four are located 0.1 mile and 70 feet lower, surrounding the large turnout and end of Anderson Landing Road.

Return the way you came.

Giving Back

The **Waddell Creek Association** manages the Rancho del Oso Nature and History Center and enriches the park through funding interpretive and research projects. Contact the association or learn more at (831) 427-2288 or www.rancho deloso.org.

Mountain Parks Foundation provides resources that expand visitors' knowledge and appreciation of the natural environment and cultural heritage of Henry Cowell and Big Basin Redwoods state parks. Contact the foundation or learn more at (831) 535-3174 or www. mountainparks.org.

Sempervirens Fund is dedicated to preserving, expanding, and linking parklands in the Santa Cruz Mountains. Contact the group or learn more at (650) 949-1453 or www.sempervirens.org.

18   Skyline-to-the-Sea Trail

RATINGS	Scenery **8** Difficulty **5** Solitude **5**
ONE-WAY DISTANCE	30 to 36 miles, depending on route
ELEVATION GAIN/LOSS	+2,500'/–5,100' to +3,800'/–6,400', depending on route
RECOMMENDED MAPS	*Castle Rock State Park Map* and *Big Basin Redwoods State Park Map* by California State Parks and *Trail Map of the Santa Cruz Mountains 1 & 2* by the Sempervirens Fund
BEST TIMES	May through October
AGENCY	Castle Rock State Park, (408) 867-2952; Big Basin Redwoods State Park, (831) 338-8860, www.bigbasin.org, www.parks.ca.gov
PERMIT	Reservations are required for Big Basin and Waterman Gap trail camps and can be made up to two months in advance by calling (831) 338-8861, Monday–Friday 10 a.m.–5 p.m.; Castle Rock Trail Camp is available on a first-come, first-served basis. Register and pay your overnight fees at the park entrance station. Big Basin trail camps are closed November through April; Castle Rock and Waterman Gap trail camps are open year-round.

Highlights

From the ridgeline spine of the Santa Cruz Mountains, the Skyline-to-the-Sea Trail descends through lush woodlands, passes sweeping vistas, lines crystalline streams, explores old-growth redwood forest, visits beautiful waterfalls, and then reaches the Pacific Ocean at Waddell Beach. It may be one of the best-known backpacking trips in the Bay Area, but the scenery and adventure are irresistibly epic.

Hike Overview

The hike begins high in the Santa Cruz Mountains in Castle Rock State Park, where spectacular views and fascinating rock formations await. From there, the journey makes a long, mostly downhill traverse through a variety of environments, from dry chaparral to lush second-growth redwood forest, en route to Big Basin Redwoods State Park. Once in the park, you travel for 8 continuous miles through magnificent old-growth

🐾 Skyline-to-the-Sea Trail

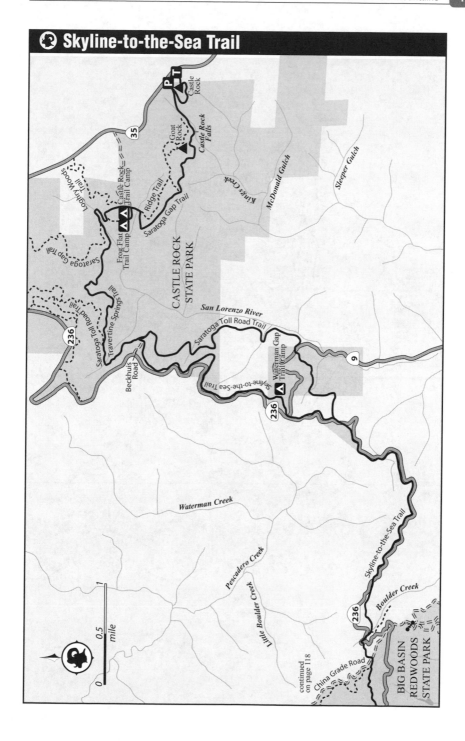

continued on page 118

♻ Skyline-to-the-Sea Trail

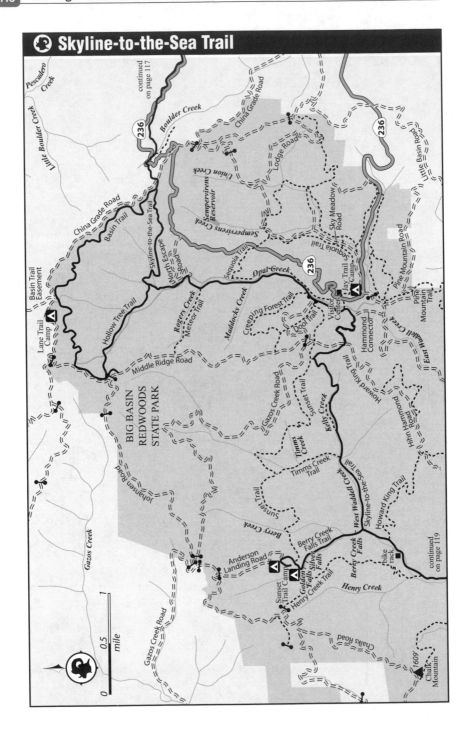

continued on page 117

continued on page 119

BIG BASIN
REDWOODS
STATE PARK

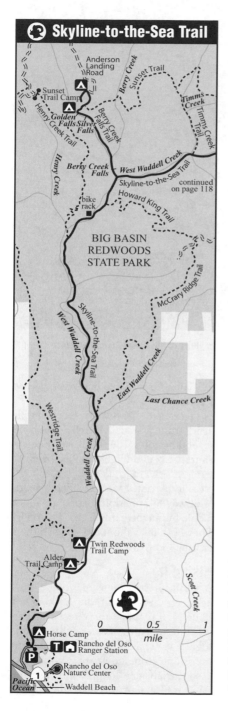

Skyline-to-the-Sea Trail

Anderson Landing Road

Sunset Trail Camp

Berry Creek
Sunset Trail

Golden Falls Silver Falls

Timms Creek

Berry Creek Falls Trail

Henry Creek Trail

Henry Creek

Berry Creek Falls
West Waddell Creek

Skyline-to-the-Sea
continued on page 118

bike rack
Howard King Trail

BIG BASIN REDWOODS STATE PARK

McCrary Ridge Trail

Skyline-to-the-Sea Trail

West Waddell Creek

East Waddell Creek

Last Chance Creek

Westridge Trail

Waddell Creek

Twin Redwoods Trail Camp

Alder Trail Camp

Scott Creek

0   0.5   1
mile

Horse Camp
Rancho del Oso Ranger Station
Rancho del Oso Nature Center
Pacific Ocean   Waddell Beach

redwood forest punctuated by tranquil streams and misting waterfalls. The final leg of the trip travels through broad Rancho del Oso canyon to reach Waddell Beach at journey's end.

It is possible to complete the journey in two long days, though three days are recommended. Spending the first night at Castle Rock Trail Camp and the second at Jay Trail Camp makes for a leisurely first day (3 miles), a long second day (16.5 miles), and a solid third day (10 miles).

Trail Camps

Seven trail camps are available for year-round overnight use. Water is available at some locations, *campfires are not allowed* (Castle Rock is an exception), and *pets are prohibited*.

Castle Rock Trail Camp is the largest and offers 20 sites spread between two adjacent areas, Main Camp and Frog Flat Camp. Campfires are permitted outside of fire season (typically December–May). **Waterman Gap Trail Camp** has six sites in a young forest near Highway 9 and 236. The sound of traffic on the nearby roads is intrusively audible. Water is usually available. **Lane Trail Camp** is accessible via a 4.2-mile detour from the main route. Six lightly used sites are available, but no water is available. **Jay Trail Camp** nestles beneath monstrous redwoods in the main visitor complex surrounding Big Basin headquarters and is situated adjacent to Highway 236. Amenities include water, hot showers in adjacent Blooms Creek Campground, and the small general store near headquarters. **Sunset Trail Camp** features 10 sites and is accessed via the fairy tale–perfect Berry Creek Falls Trail, a 1.2-mile detour off the main route. Berry Creek is a third of a mile away and provides water. **Twin Redwoods Trail Camp** sits

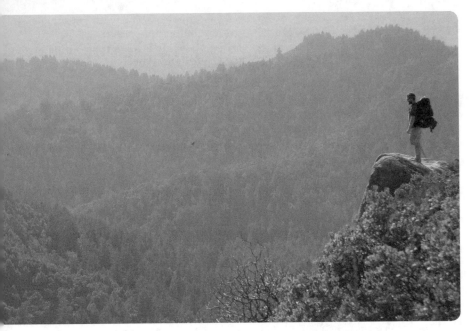

A backpacker on the Skyline-to-the-Sea Trail enjoys views of the Santa Cruz Mountains.

in a shady copse of giant bay trees adjacent to Waddell Creek. **Alder Trail Camp** is tucked among young alders near Waddell Creek.

Getting There

To reach the trailhead at Castle Rock State Park, take Highway 35 south of the Highway 9 junction for 2.5 miles; the posted entrance is located on the west side of the road.

To reach the trailhead at Waddell Beach, take Highway 1 to Waddell Beach, located 4.0 miles north of Davenport. Turn inland at the closed (but unlocked) gate found north of Waddell Creek, and follow the road 0.5 mile to the Rancho del Oso Ranger Station and parking lot. Public transportation is available to Waddell Beach from downtown Santa Cruz twice daily with the Santa Cruz Metro bus service (**www. scmtd.com**).

To reach the Castle Rock Trailhead from Waddell Beach, you have several options. The southern route via Santa Cruz and Highway 9 is the most straightforward and easy to follow. Northern routes via Pescadero Road, Highway 84, or Alpine Road are more scenic but involve much twistier roads. They both take about the same amount of time (60 to 90 minutes).

Hiking It

A small forest of signs marks the trailhead at the edge of the parking lot (0.0/3,070'). While the direct route to the trail camp proceeds straight on Saratoga Gap Trail, the park's fascinating sandstone formations are accessed via a short half-mile loop that rejoins the main trail a short distance ahead. It is an attraction well worth visiting—those arriving late in the day should consider exploring this area on the return trip.

To begin among the boulders, bear left at the trailhead toward Castle Rock, turn right on the immediate fire road, and quickly reach the first wild stone pile on the left. From here interlaced paths wind past a variety of outcrops before reaching Castle Rock itself, an apartment-sized monolith deeply gouged by erosion. After exploring this unusual geologic world, proceed the short distance to Saratoga Gap Trail and bear left.

To head directly to the campground from the trailhead (0.0/3,070'), proceed straight on Saratoga Gap Trail as it passes through a mixed-evergreen forest dominated by the drooping evergreen branches of Douglas-fir, the large spiny leaves of tanoak, and the twisting trunks of madrone. A trailside understory of blackberry and poison oak discourages a departure from the soft path as it begins its descent into the Kings Creek drainage, one of the uppermost headwaters of the San Lorenzo River.

Dropping into a dry gully, the trail quickly passes a junction on the left for Castle Rock (0.1/3,000') where those exploring the sandstone formations rejoin the main trail. The trail continues downward and a spring soon appears, feeding Kings Creek as the broad leaves of bigleaf maple appear overhead and thick clumps of sword ferns sprout along the moist creek bed. Crossing the creek, the trail reaches the junction with Ridge Trail (0.5/2,730') Continue straight on Saratoga Gap Trail.

A few young redwoods join large Douglas-firs as Saratoga Gap Trail continues briefly along the creek to reach the sheer overlook for the thin cascade of Castle Rock Falls (0.7/2,700'). From

here Kings Creek plummets downward and drops more than a thousand vertical feet in less than a mile. Heading away from the creek, Saratoga Gap Trail quickly passes onto drier slopes where coffee berry, toyon, and fragrant California bay appear—plants better adapted to a world of less moisture.

The hike traverses steep slopes, passing through a world of chaparral protruded by sandstone boulders, and enters a stand of rustling black oaks shortly before reaching a connector trail on the right leading to nearby Ridge Trail (1.5/2,560'). Continue straight on Saratoga Gap Trail as spectacular views soon open into the heart of the Santa Cruz Mountains.

Looking south beyond the vast drainage of the San Lorenzo River, the Monterey peninsula can be identified across Monterey Bay on clear days (a distance of more than 40 miles). To the west, the low ridge separating the San Lorenzo River and Pescadero Creek watersheds is apparent; the Skyline-to-the-Sea Trail follows this divide en route to Big Basin Redwoods State Park. Tall Bonny Doon Ridge hems the San Lorenzo River to the southwest, while Butano Ridge rises above Pescadero Creek to the west. The deep canyon of Pescadero Creek curves out-of-sight to the northwest, harboring many an overnight outdoor adventure in its recesses—Portola Redwoods State Park, Memorial County Park, and Pescadero Creek County Park all await exploration.

Now gradually descending, you pass through chaparral thick with coyote brush and poison oak. Narrow and rocky in places, the trail winds along sheer slopes before turning sharply right to pass through a suddenly thick forest of tanoak and madrone before reaching the junction with Ridge Trail

(2.5/2,400'). To reach the trail camp, bear left, and then left again on the wide fire road to reach the main area (2.7/2,400'). Knobcone pines abruptly appear beside young Douglas-firs in this section, their twisted architecture and namesake cones making them easy to identify. The 15 sites of the Main Camp area are located nearby off Saratoga Gap Trail, while the 5 sites of more-removed Frog Flat Camp are located a quarter mile downhill on Service Road Trail, just below the intersection with Frog Flat Trail.

From the Main Camp, continue on wide Saratoga Gap Trail as it descends to quickly pass Frog Flat Trail on the left (3.0/2,240') and enters the moist environment of Craig Springs Creek. You cross the small stream, then rise quickly to reach Travertine Springs Trail (3.4/2,100'). Bear left on wide Travertine Springs Trail to parallel the stream, noting the small redwood trees that appear here for the first time.

The trail curves away from the stream, which abruptly drops out-of-sight below, and narrows before dropping into a lush environment of chain ferns and small dogwood trees. You continue a steady descent through shady woods; a pair of switchbacks soon deposit you at the most significant waterway yet—the headwaters of the

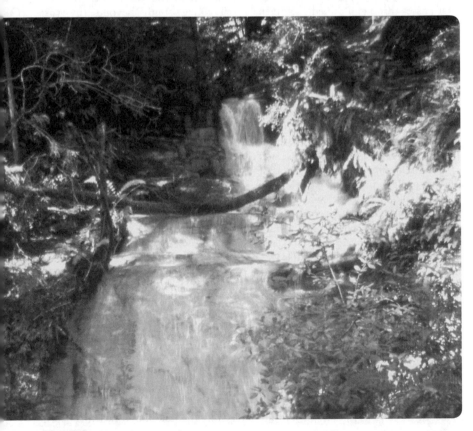

Silver Falls

San Lorenzo River itself (4.4/1,680'). Stout Douglas-firs line the stream.

From here, an undulating traverse provides intermittent views of the San Lorenzo watershed en route to Travertine Springs (5.2/1,760'), where a striking patch of large equisetum, or horsetail, flourishes beneath an enormous, six-trunked bay tree. A fenced-off area protects the extensive fen and spring, though a thin streamlet usually provides a trickle sufficient for obtaining water.

Continuing, you traverse steadily to reach the junction with Saratoga Toll Road Trail (5.5/1,800'). Bear left and follow Saratoga Toll Road Trail on an easy descent through open mixed-evergreen woods, crossing the watershed of ephemeral Tin Can Creek and then curving left above a deepening gorge to reach Beckhuis Road Trail (6.3/1,550').

If you are staying at Waterman Gap Trail Camp, your most direct option is to bear right on Beckhuis Road Trail for 0.2 mile, left on Cutoff Trail for 0.2 mile, and then left for 2.6 miles along the Skyline-to-the-Sea Trail parallel to Highway 9. The next day, remain on the Skyline-to-the-Sea Trail for another mile to reach the continuing route at the junction with Saratoga Toll Road Trail.

Otherwise remain on Saratoga Toll Road Trail, bearing right at the immediate fork to follow the wide trail on a fast, easy downhill traverse. Along the way you abruptly encounter some large redwoods in a significant grove; fire scars on their trunks tell the story of redwoods' flame-resistant bark. The trail then winds through second-growth redwood forest, crosses beneath power lines, and then curves into and around a deeper drainage. You next encounter a gated fire road on the left leading down to the nearby

San Lorenzo River, and then quickly reach the Skyline-to-the-Sea Interconnector Trail (9.5/800').

Turn right on single-track Interconnector Trail, climbing steeply through redwood forest to immediately reach a jarring encounter with the pavement and traffic of Highway 9 (9.7/910'). The trail crosses the highway, continues over a small ridgeline, and then drops along a drier south-facing slope before reentering redwood forest. After crossing a dry streambed, you climb via several closely-spaced switchbacks and pass the largest redwood yet—a fire-scarred specimen, its trunk hollowed out by flame. The route crosses and recrosses a power line corridor, then runs along a ridgeline before making a final steep boost to reach the Skyline-to-the-Sea Trail by Highway 236 (11.4/1,300').

Turning left, you now follow alongside Highway 236 for several undulating miles through dense second-growth redwood forest, crossing several private roads en route. After crossing Highway 236 (14.7/1,900'), the hike finally curves away from the road. Big Basin Redwoods State Park is only a short distance ahead.

The park boundary is not marked, but the transition is readily apparent as several old-growth trees appear along the trail. The trail leads past East Ridge Trail on the left by trickling Boulder Creek (15.4/1,780'), then turns uphill to cross Highway 236 yet again (15.5/1,820'). You climb out of the San Lorenzo River watershed and cross paved China Grade Road (16.0/1,980'), where the flora abruptly changes to dry chaparral marked by the presence of coyote brush, toyon, yerba santa, buck brush, and canyon live oaks. Excellent views look toward the southwest, including the deep drainage of Waddell Creek and the still-distant Pacific Ocean. Past the road, the trail quickly encounters Basin Trail on the right (16.1/1,980'). (Hikers continuing on the Skyline-to-the-Sea Trail can skip the following description to Lane Trail Camp.)

SIDE TRIP TO LANE TRAIL CAMP
Lane Trail Camp offers six campsites in a dense forest of tanoak in one of Big Basin's least visited areas. A 6-mile loop follows the Basin Trail to the campsites and then returns to the main route via the Hollow Tree Trail. Rejoining the Skyline-to-the-Sea Trail 1.8 miles past the Basin Trail junction, this variation adds 4.2 miles and 700 feet of elevation gain and loss to the overall journey. Water is *not* available anywhere in the vicinity. The last reli-

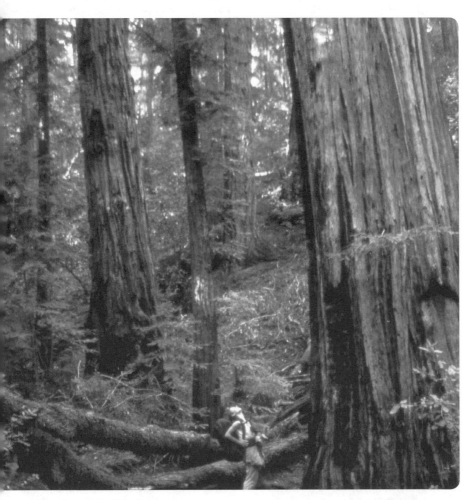

Vast forest of redwoods enormous

able source is at Waterman Gap Trail Camp, though a few ephemeral trickles can be found along Basin Trail during wet periods.

From the junction with the Skyline-to-the-Sea Trail (0.0/1,960'), Basin Trail begins an undulating, gradually rising traverse along the uppermost slopes of the Waddell Creek watershed. After passing several of the many excellent viewpoints found along this section, the trail enters the shade of dense madrone trees and continues through a more diverse mixed-evergreen forest of Douglas-fir, tanoak, coast live oak, and the occasional redwood. Cresting a small rise, the trail then curves right and enters a region marked in recent years by wildfire.

Flame-blackened trunks of gnarled redwoods emerge from the hillside before the trail returns to south-facing slopes and a drier world dominated by knobcone pines. A spindly conifer with namesake cones bursting from everywhere (including on branches and trunks), knobcone pines survive through a process called serotiny—their cones open only during wildfire. Freshly opened cones populate the burned-out, nutrient-rich soil with a massive influx of seeds, resulting in a region dominated by young trees. As the trail passes through this unusual forest, chaparral species such as manzanita and sticky monkeyflower can be found intermixed in the dry environment.

Undulating slowly upward the trail next winds through unusual sandstone outcrops before returning to shady north-facing slopes where redwoods instantly reappear. The trail passes three small ephemeral creeks, then turns abruptly uphill to follow a narrow creek gully to reach a four-way junction (3.1/2,280'). Hollow Tree Trail—your continuing route—goes

left, but Lane Trail Camp is straight ahead, a short 0.1 mile from this junction on a narrow, slightly overgrown trail. A right turn at the junction takes you to China Grade Road and the start of the Basin Trail Easement, which connects Portola Redwoods and Big Basin Redwoods state parks.

The return descent on Hollow Tree Trail winds through thick vegetation regenerating from the recent wildfire—blackened young redwoods less than a foot in diameter indicate how recently the area charred. A few old-growth redwood survivors appear intermittently as well, demonstrating their resistance to wildfire with burn marks more than 30 feet off the ground. The trail's final view soon opens up, looking down the drainage of Opal Creek and the direction of descent.

You cross the Opal Creek headwaters by a massive redwood tree and end the contouring traverse by the large metal detritus of Johansen Shingle Mill (built in 1927). Massive boilers and large metal pieces can be explored just off the trail. The trail next drops steeply down the narrow creek gully and quickly reaches a short connector trail leading to Middle Ridge Fire Road (4.6/1,780'). Bearing left, the trail continues its steep descent, makes two creek crossings, and then parallels the flowing stream as it babbles among moss-coated boulders. Crossing yet another small tributary, the trail contours through a lush forest before rejoining the Skyline-to-the Sea Trail (6.0/1,270'). Bear right and follow the description below.

From the junction with the Basin Trail (16.1/1,980'), the Skyline-to-the-Sea Trail continues through dense chaparral punctuated by spindly knobcone pines—enjoy the hike's final views as you traverse the slopes. The route then turns downhill, curves right to reenter lush redwood forest, and crosses two small headwater trickles of Opal Creek shortly before the Hollow Tree Trail enters from the right (17.9/1,270').

Let the glory begin! For the next 8 miles, the hike remains entirely within magnificent old-growth redwood forest. You cross Opal Creek on a wooden walkway and follow the burbling stream past large chain ferns and humongous redwoods. You next reach paved North Escape Road near an informative kiosk (18.4/1,060'). Cross Opal Creek on the paved bridge, then immediately bear right to return to the trail, which briefly parallels the road, momentarily rejoins it, and then passes Meteor Trail on the right (18.6/1,070'). The route touches the road again at another bridge crossing (18.9/1,040'). Sequoia Trail continues on the opposite side, but the Skyline-to-the-Sea Trail leaves the road at this point to remain on the right (west) side of Opal Creek.

Cruising close to the water past the fluted trunks of giant redwoods, the trail next reaches Maddocks Creek, where an interpretive placard tells the story of an early settler who built an entire cabin from a single redwood tree. Look for the soft leaves of hazel bushes as you continue on the muddy trail, pass Creeping Forest Trail (19.8/970') and Gazos Creek Road (19.9/970'), and then reach Dool Trail on the right (20.0/960'), named for the third park warden of Big Basin Redwoods State Park. Continue straight to quickly reach the junction for the Big Basin headquarters area on the left (20.4/950'). To reach Jay Trail Camp and the park visitor center (plus the goodies at the park's small general store), turn left here to cross Opal Creek. Jay Trail Camp is located a quarter mile south

of park headquarters on the north side of the highway.

The continuing hike on the Skyline-to-the-Sea Trail quickly passes the Hammond Connector on the left (20.4/970') and begins a steady climb out of the East Waddell Creek drainage. After several switchbacks, the trail crests into the West Waddell Creek drainage at the junction with Howard King Trail (21.1/1,320').

Continuing straight, you pass a connector to Sunset Trail on the right (21.5/1,170') and rapidly descend though spectacular old-growth redwood forest—dozens of perfect trees fill the forest in every direction. A bridge soon leads across Kelly Creek, where an alternate route splits right and runs along the stream before rejoining the main trail 0.4 mile later. Past Timms Creek Trail (22.8/530'), the canyon narrows and becomes rockier. The trail drops to cross West Waddell Creek, briefly climbs to a tantalizing view of Berry Creek Falls, and then descends to reach Berry Creek Falls Trail (24.2/350') at the confluence of the two creeks.

SIDE TRIP TO BERRY CREEK FALLS AND SUNSET TRAIL CAMP　Even if you're not staying at Sunset Trail Camp, drop your pack here and make the brief side trip to Berry Creek Falls. Berry Creek Falls Trail immediately leads to a large viewing platform for the waterfall, a misty cascade that nourishes lush surrounding greenery. Thimbleberry and sword fern coat the damp ground below, tanoak and redwoods rise above, and five-finger ferns wave from the surrounding steep, mossy slopes.

The continuing trail climbs steeply above the falls and crosses Berry Creek, staying close to the water in a fairytale world of giant trees. The muddy path next reaches Silver Falls, climbing above it via a steep cable-protected section to reach Golden Falls, a series of cascades that slide over brilliant orange sandstone. The trail then curves right to climb out of the narrow creek canyon and reach Sunset Trail. To reach Sunset Trail Camp, turn left and ascend the narrow trail to Anderson Landing Road in 0.2 mile. Six sites are available directly across the road (follow the signs); four more are located 0.1 mile and 70 feet lower around a large turnout.

From the Berry Creek Falls Trail (24.2/350'), the Skyline-to-the-Sea Trail descends to cross rushing West Waddell Creek on a seasonal bridge. Arcing

bigleaf maples overhead provide ideal hunting grounds for spiders, which trap insects flying up the open creek corridor. Dozens of perfect webs are everywhere, their strands glistening with the moisture of fog and rain. Past this point, the trail widens to become a fire road and the forest immediately transforms into denser, younger second-growth. The route follows the wide and level fire road for the remainder of the hike.

The trail passes Howard King Trail on the left (24.5/350'), then recrosses the creek and encounters a bike rack. Crossing the stream one last time, the trail passes a few old-growth trees, momentarily narrows to avoid a large

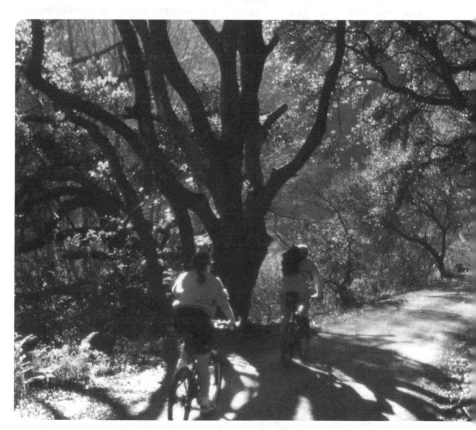

Biking inland from the sea

washout, and reaches Henry Creek Trail on the right (25.1/300'). The canyon broadens and members of the approaching coastal scrub community start to appear: ceanothus, sticky monkeyflower, coyote brush, coffee berry, blackberry tangles, poison oak, and stinging nettle. The trail slowly descends to McCrary Ridge Trail on the left (27.4/100'), crosses East Waddell Creek on a metal bridge, and reaches the former site of Camp Herbert (27.5/100').

Past Camp Herbert, the trail runs along the boundary between parkland and gated private property. Redwoods become increasingly scarce and poison oak explodes in abundance. Soon the large, two-headed redwood tree that gives Twin Redwoods Trail Camp its name appears (28.4/60'). Continuing, the Skyline-to-the-Sea Trail quickly passes Clark Connection Trail on the right, which leads to an alternate, hikers-only route back to Rancho del Oso Ranger Station. To take this narrower, less-traveled trail, bear right to cross Waddell Creek and then turn left downstream (Clark Connection Trail continues upslope). The path climbs briefly and contours along the slopes, crossing several small creeks. Enjoy a few intermittent views of the area—including a glimpse of the Pacific Ocean—before descending to reach Rancho del Oso Ranger Station.

If you remain on the easier road, you quickly reach Alder Trail Camp on the right (28.6/40') and then pass through the hike's final redwood grove. Here lurks a huge and gnarled speci-men known as the Eagle Tree, spared the logging ax because of its contorted shape. The broad trail widens as it passes a gated private road on the left, then crosses Waddell Creek one last time, and passes through a section of private property—please stay on the road. You pass another private road shortly before reaching Horse Camp and the Rancho del Oso Ranger Station (29.6/20'). The hike's final journey to the beach follows the paved road from the parking area to the unlocked gate by Highway 1. Cross the busy road to reach the sandy expanse of Waddell Beach and your journey's end (30.1/0').

Giving Back

Portola and Castle Rock Foundation supports interpretive projects at Portola Redwoods and Castle Rock state parks and publishes maps, brochures, and interpretive materials for the parks. Contact the foundation or learn more at (650) 948-9098 or **www.parks.ca.gov/ default.asp?page_id=22075**.

Mountain Parks Foundation provides resources that expand visitors' knowledge and appreciation of the natural environment and cultural heritage of Henry Cowell and Big Basin Redwoods state parks. Contact the foundation or learn more at (831) 535-3174 or **www. mountainparks.org**.

Sempervirens Fund is dedicated to preserving, expanding, and linking parklands in the Santa Cruz Mountains. Contact the group or learn more about them at (650) 949-1453 or **www. sempervirens.org**.

East of the Bay

Fantastic oaks twist skyward from hillsides flush with the Bay Area's most prolific wildflower displays. The open landscape reveals ever-changing views of seemingly endless valleys and ridgelines. Wildlife thrives in this remote and hilly country, where extensive opportunities for solitude and adventure await the intrepid hiker.

For the purposes of this book, East of the Bay includes the ecologically similar regions found east of San Francisco Bay and the Santa Clara Valley. A multitude of north-south trending ridges compose the hilly terrain, offering little in the way of level ground. In the northern area, monolithic Mt. Diablo dominates; at 3,849 feet it towers over the surrounding landscape and overlooks the lower-lying Oakland and Berkeley Hills to the west. Farther south, the land is wrinkled into the tortured Diablo Range, a series of furrowed ridges and peaks rising 3,000 feet and higher.

Backpacking trips are largely confined to two destinations: Henry W. Coe State Park and the Ohlone Trail, which spans Mission Peak Regional Preserve, Sunol Regional Wilderness, Ohlone Regional Wilderness, and Del Valle Regional Park. Both offer opportunities to explore the Bay Area's deepest backcountry on extended multiday excursions, as well as on shorter, overnight trips. The only other backpacking option is Black Diamond Mines Regional Preserve, a place of rich history, woodlands, and wildlife in the eastern Mt. Diablo foothills.

19 Black Diamond Mines Regional Preserve

RATINGS	Scenery **7** Difficulty **5** Solitude **4**
ROUND-TRIP DISTANCE	6.8 miles
ELEVATION GAIN/LOSS	+1,700'/–1,700'
OPTIONAL MAP	*Black Diamond Mines Regional Preserve Map* by the East Bay Regional Park District
BEST TIMES	Spring and fall
AGENCY	Black Diamond Mines Regional Preserve, (510) 544-2750, **www. ebparks.org/parks/black-diamond**. Visitor center is open on weekends (spring through fall) 10 a.m.–4:30 p.m. and on weekdays as staffing allows.
PERMIT	Trail camp reservations ($5 per person, plus a one-time $8 reservation fee) can be made for the entire calendar year beginning February 1. Call 888-EBPARKS (327-2757), 8:30 a.m.–4 p.m. Monday–Friday. Campers can make last-minute arrangements at the park if space is available.

Highlights

Hike through history as you enjoy expansive views of cow-studded hills, twisting oaks, radiant wildflowers, and abundant wildlife.

Hike Overview

This easy loop winds along fire roads and single-track trails through pleasant oak woodlands that seasonally burst with wildflowers (March–May). The park also bursts with an abundance of cows year-round, though wildlife is commonly seen darting beneath and above the open woodlands. Cows still seem to own the place, however, and it's you—not them—that are fenced in at night. Dogs are allowed and may run unleashed in the backcountry if under voice control. Avoid the wettest times of year; conditions can be unpleasantly muddy. Skip summer as well, when heat sears the many un-shaded miles of trail.

Trail Camp

A small, fenced enclosure protects **Stewartville Backpack Camp**, situated at valley bottom very near the former coal-mining town of Stewartville. Two picnic tables and a few level tent sites are available beneath the shady boughs of buckeye, olive, and walnut trees (the latter two introduced by miners). Cows roam freely about the area, but a sense of isolation from today's world permeates the site. The trail camp is single-occupancy (only one group may use it at a time), and is reserved well in advance for spring and fall weekends.

Residents of Alameda and Contra Costa counties can make reservations beginning November 1 for the entire following calendar year. If the site is not reserved, it is available on a first-come, first-served basis—call ahead to check.

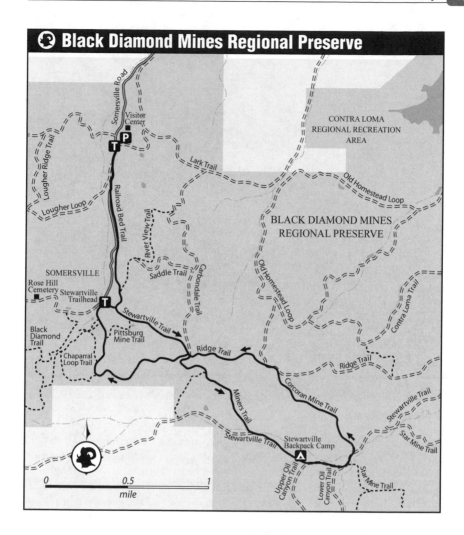

Black Diamond Mines Regional Preserve

Getting There

Take the Somersville exit from Highway 4 in Antioch and proceed south on Somersville Road for 2.6 miles to reach park headquarters on the left. Backpackers are required to leave their vehicles in the headquarters parking lot. However, you can avoid a mile of walking with full packs by dropping equipment off at the Stewartville Trailhead a mile farther at road's end.

Hiking It

The following describes the most direct route to the backpack camp, returning via a slightly longer route that visits scenic views and several interesting sites. From the headquarters parking lot (0.0/500'), proceed south along Railroad Bed Trail toward the Stewartville Trailhead. Wide Railroad Bed Trail parallels the road, then slowly gains elevation as it follows the old

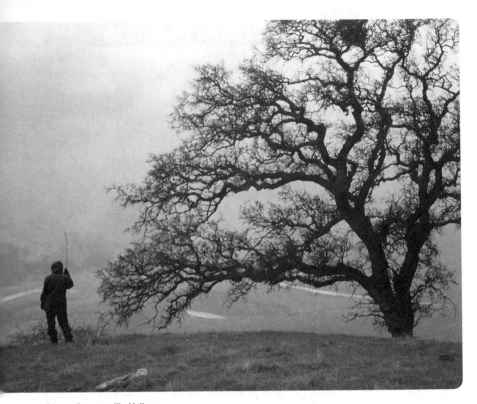

Above Stewartville Valley

route of the Pittsburg Railroad. Built in the 1860s and operating until the early 1900s, the railroad transported coal 5 miles from the Somersville area to Pittsburg Landing on the Sacramento River for shipment.

Bear left at the junction with Stewartville Trail (0.8/800'). (If you are starting your hike from road's end at the backpack drop-off point, continue straight on the paved road for 100 yards, and bear left on Stewartville Trail to quickly reach the junction with Railroad Bed Trail.)

Memories of mining days are evident on the opposite valley slopes to the west, where Rose Hill Cemetery houses the remains of local Protestants who succumbed to mine disasters and epidemics. Local flora includes twisting blue oaks laden with large tangles of mistletoe, wispy gray pines with massive cones, and the evergreen leaves of interior live oak. Numerous introduced species of trees also are abundant in this area, including Tree of Heaven, easily identified by its clusters of papery shaker seed pods; California pepper tree, an evergreen with narrow leaves seasonally dangling with small red berries; and eucalyptus.

Continue on wide Stewartville Trail straight past Pittsburg Mine Trail junction as the path steadily climbs above Markley Canyon to reach the ridgetop and junction with Ridge and

Carbondale trails (1.4/1,150'). Continue straight through the gate to reach a second junction with Ridge Trail on the left (your return route), and bear right to remain on Stewartville Trail. Winding gradually down into the broad valley, the trail shortly reaches the junction with Miners Trail (1.8/980').

Follow Miners Trail as it traverses above the valley alongside manzanita, chamise, toyon, interior and coast live oaks, and gray pines. To the southwest, Mt. Diablo (3849') can be seen looming over the land a scant 6 miles away. Miners Trail then plummets down to the valley floor and passes above the old entrance to Central Mine, which operated for nearly 40 years during the late 19th century. At valley bottom

(2.5/550'), proceed across the stream gully to return to Stewartville Trail, and bear left to reach the backpack camp (3.0/500').

To return to the trailhead, continue on Stewartville Trail past three intersections on the right—for Upper and Lower Oil Canyon trails and Star Mine Trail—to reach the junction with Corcoran Mine Trail (3.3/460'). Bear left and begin climbing wide Corcoran Mine Trail past sandstone outcrops, large manzanita bushes, and gray pines. Blue oaks begin to dominate and views get ever nicer as the route climbs to the junction with Ridge Trail (4.1/1,100'). Continue left on Ridge Trail and pass a junction on the right for Acorn Trail (4.2/1,140'), where far-reaching views

BLACK DIAMONDS

Once upon a time—50 million years or so ago—the marshy edge of California was in today's nearby town of Antioch. Towering volcanoes loomed to the east where the Sierra Nevada now rise, their flanks rolling down to a broad coastal plain. To the west was the deep blue sea. Creatures and plants forgotten by time lived and died here, flourishing in an equitable climate by the sea. As the sea level rose and fell in its eternal cycle of flux, their remains were buried by sand and mud. And coal they became, black diamonds of fortune upon which towns would appear in the human future.

The coal became exposed at the surface as tectonic activity wrinkled Mt. Diablo and its surroundings upward during the past 2 to 3 million years. Rare was this band of coal and pressing were the energy needs of the blossoming city of San Francisco. The beds quickly became the site of California's largest coal mining operation in the years following the Gold Rush; from the 1860s to the turn of the century, five boomtowns supported hundreds of miners and their families. In the early 1900s the operation was abandoned as cheaper coal became available elsewhere and oil appeared on the fossil fuel scene. Two of these former townsites—Somersville and Stewartsville—are visited on this hike. If you are interested in a more hands-on exploration of the region's mining history, underground tours of Hazel Atlas Mine are offered on weekends from March through November. Contact the park for more information and a current schedule.

to the northeast reveal the confluence of the mighty Sacramento and San Joaquin rivers and their broad, fanning delta; views southwest are dominated by the massif of Mt. Diablo.

Returning to the earlier junctions with Stewartville Trail (4.7/1,150'), you can head back to the trailhead on a different—and interesting—route by remaining on Ridge Trail as it continues west. Oaks disappear as Ridge Trail passes through a chaparral community of chamise and manzanita joined for the first time by Coulter pines, a less common tree here at the northern limits of its range. Producing the largest cones of any conifer, it can be identi-

fied by its erect, single-trunk character and long needles in bundles of three. A maze of trails winds through the area; bear right at the junction with Chaparral Loop (5.4/1,130'), and remain right at all junctions for the most direct route down to Stewartville Trailhead (5.8/760'). Along the way you pass numerous artifacts from mining days, including the entrance to Hazel Atlas Mine (see sidebar, page 133). Return to the headquarters parking lot on Railroad Bed Trail (6.8/500').

Giving Back

The **Regional Parks Foundation** supports and funds the acquisition, devel-

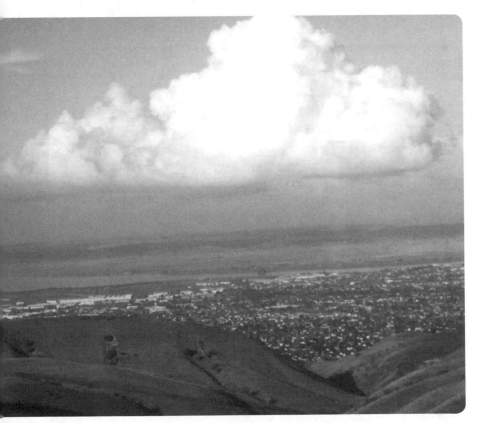

Cloud over humanity, looking north to Antioch

opment, and stewardship of parklands in the East Bay Regional Park District through private contributions. Contact the foundation or learn more at (510) 544-2200 or **www.regionalparks foundation.org.**

Anyone interested in volunteering for Black Diamond Mines Regional Preserve—or any other unit of the **East Bay Regional Park District**—can contact the district's volunteer coordinator for more information at (510) 544-2515 or volunteers@ebparks.org.

20 Mission Peak Regional Preserve Loop

RATINGS	Scenery **9** Difficulty **6** Solitude **2**
ROUND-TRIP DISTANCE	6.4 miles
ELEVATION GAIN/LOSS	+2,000'/–2,000'
RECOMMENDED MAPS	*Mission Peak Regional Preserve Map* and *Ohlone Wilderness Regional Trail Permit and Map,* both by the East Bay Regional Park District
BEST TIMES	Year-round
AGENCY	Mission Peak Regional Preserve, (510) 544-3246, **www.ebparks.org/ parks/mission**
PERMIT	Trail camp reservations ($5 per person, plus a one-time $8 reservation fee) are required and can be made for the entire calendar year beginning February 1. Call 888-EBPARKS (327-2757), 8:30 a.m.–4 p.m. Monday–Friday.

Highlights
A quiet trail camp hides behind the soaring summit of landmark Mission Peak. Secluded high above the Bay Area yet hidden from its bustle, it offers a tranquil destination with superlative views along the way.

Trail Camp
Eagle Spring Backpack Camp is situated on the east side of Mission Peak, perched just below the summit at 2,200 feet. Four sites are available. Three are exposed with no shade or wind protection, the fourth sits beneath the shady boughs of a large bay tree. Each has its own picnic table. The camp is fenced

to keep out the many roving bovines; a water pump and outhouse are available. Excellent views look east into the oak-studded wilds of the Diablo Range. Note that residents of Alameda and Contra Costa counties can make reservations early, beginning November 1 for the entire following year. *Fires, dogs, and bicycles are prohibited.*

Getting There
Take I-680 to Fremont. From northbound I-680, take the Mission Boulevard exit and proceed straight on Mission Boulevard 0.7 mile. Turn right on Stanford Avenue and proceed 0.6 mile to the parking lot and trailhead. From

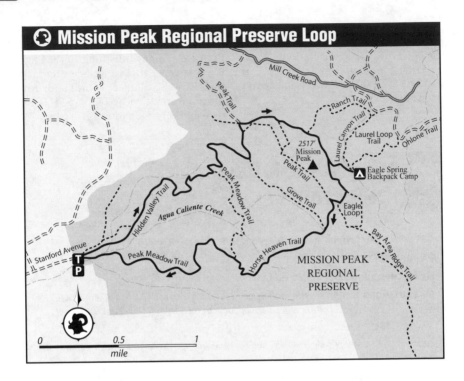

Mission Peak Regional Preserve Loop

southbound p680, take the exit for Mission Boulevard and Highway 238, turn left on Mission Boulevard, go 2.8 miles, turn left on Stanford Avenue, and proceed as above.

Public transportation is possible— AC Transit #217 runs from the Fremont BART Station to Stanford Avenue and Mission Boulevard. Learn more about schedules and services at (510) 817-1717 or www.actransit.org.

Hiking It

Your journey begins at the gate (0.0/410') on a wide fire road. The entire western flank of Mission Peak rises before you, laced by the watershed of Agua Caliente Creek. Cattle browse the grassy hillsides. Ohlone Trail signpost 1 quickly appears, the first of many numbered postings listed on the

Ohlone Wilderness Regional Trail Permit and Map. The trail passes through numerous gates; leave them as you find them.

Continue straight as Peak Meadow Trail forks to the right (0.2/470'). Your wide path curves left toward more open views, passing a copse of coast live oak on the right. Look for buckeye and sycamore trees in the small nearby creek gully. The trail bears right to cross this small drainage, then curves and briefly parallels Agua Caliente Creek. You next cross a cattle guard and enter the fenced-off world of cattle country. Looking behind you to the west, Coyote Hills dimple the horizon beyond Fremont.

Now steadily climbing, you curve upward to attain a discernible ridgeline. As you crest beyond 1,000 feet in elevation, the trail briefly eases to pass the first of several benches overlooking the South Bay and the East of the Bay beyond. The sustained ascent next passes Peak Meadow Trail on the right (1.5/1,490') and reaches a cattle guard below the rocky ramparts of the summit massif. Large sandstone (graywacke) boulders rest on the slopes, a lone coast live oak holds a tenuous foothold below, and a park residence is visible ahead in the distance across the meadow.

Bear left at the next junction with Grove Trail (2.2/1,810') to quickly reach another junction (2.4/1,990')—go right on the rougher and more rutted road. At signpost 4 (2.5/2,060'), views north open up toward Mount Diablo and the East Bay Hills as you round the shoulder of Mission Peak. Continuing right on Eagle Trail, you soon encounter a junction with Peak Trail (2.7/2,130') and attain your first views east into the hills of Sunol Regional Wilderness and Ohlone Regional Wilderness (and Trail) beyond. Remain on Eagle Trail as it traverses down to reach signpost 6 at 2,050 (2.9/2,050') and then the trail camp (3.0/2,200').

The summit is within easy striking distance from camp; fully survey it on a 1.7-mile loop via Eagle and Peak trails (elevation gain and loss of +550'/-550'). The loop can be completed in either direction; clockwise is recommended. A unique pipe viewer on the summit identifies distant landmarks; you can see San Francisco, Mount Tamalpais, the East of the Bay, and the entire South Bay.

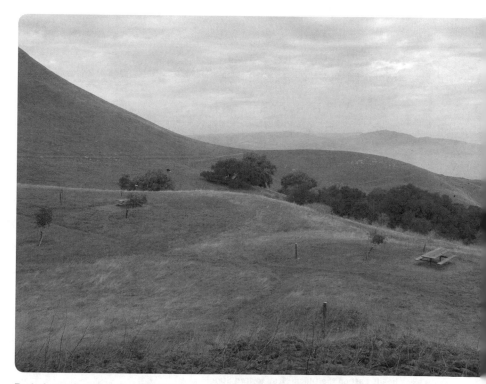

Eagle Spring Backpack Camp offers views east into the Ohlone Wilderness.

To return to the trailhead, you have two options. Return the way you came (easiest, shortest option) or complete a loop via Horse Heaven and Peak Meadow trails. To complete the loop, continue south from camp and bear right toward the summit ridge on the obvious path (3.3/2,200'). Once you reach the low saddle in the ridge (3.4/2,300'), continue left and downhill on Horse Heaven Trail.

You quickly pass Peak Meadow Trail on the right (3.6/2,160') and then begin a steep, sustained, and view-rich descent to eventually reach the junction with Peak Meadow Trail (5.1/1,400'). Continue straight on Peak Meadow Trail as it makes the final drop down the mountainside to return you to the trailhead area (6.4/410').

Giving Back

The **Regional Parks Foundation** supports and funds the acquisition, development, and stewardship of parklands in the East Bay Regional Park District through private contributions. Contact the foundation or learn more at (510) 544-2200 or **www.regionalparksfoundation.org.**

Anyone interested in volunteering for Mission Peak Regional Preserve— or any other unit of the **East Bay Regional Park District**—can contact the district's volunteer coordinator for more information at (510) 544-2515 or volunteers@ebparks.org.

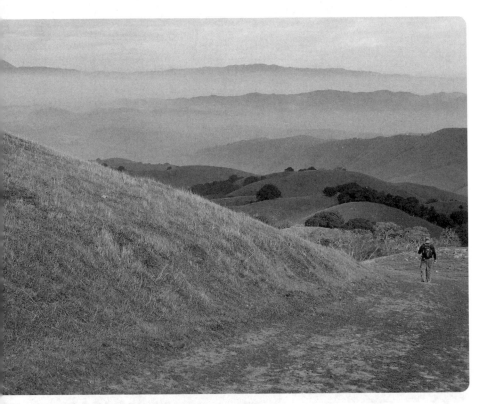

A hiker heads east on the Ohlone Trail toward Sunol.

21 Sunol Regional Wilderness:
SUNOL BACKPACK CAMP LOOP

RATINGS	Scenery **8** Difficulty **6** Solitude **7**
ROUND-TRIP DISTANCE	5.9 miles
ELEVATION GAIN/LOSS	+1,100'/–1,100'
RECOMMENDED MAPS	*Sunol Regional Wilderness Park Map* and *Ohlone Wilderness Regional Trail Permit and Map*, both by the East Bay Regional Park District
BEST TIMES	February through May
AGENCY	Sunol Regional Wilderness, (510) 544-3249, **www.ebparks.org/ parks/sunol**. Park visitor center is open 10 a.m.–5 p.m. on weekends in summer and intermittently on weekends the rest of the year.
PERMIT	Trail camp reservations ($5 per person, plus a one-time $8 reservation fee) can be made for the entire calendar year beginning February 1. Call 888-EBPARKS (327-2757), 8:30 a.m.–4 p.m. Monday–Friday. Campers can make last-minute arrangements at the park if space is available.

Highlights

Shielded from view behind landmark Mission Peak, peaceful Sunol Wilderness offers escape in beautiful rolling woodlands. An idyllic backcountry camping area at the hike's midpoint provides a tranquil setting and far-reaching views for an overnight stay.

Hike Overview

Explore the multifaceted character of Sunol Wilderness as you climb through majestic oak woodlands, walk open hillsides, and pause at substantial Alameda Creek as it rushes through a scenic section dubbed "Little Yosemite." This loop hike can be completed year-round, but spring is the time to come as hillsides are carpeted green and wildflowers explode in one of the Bay Area's most dazzling and diverse displays. Cows graze throughout the park, creating a pleasant manicured landscape full of cowpie minefields. Water is available at the trailhead.

Trail Camp

Sunol Backpack Camp offers seven sites scattered across 500 vertical feet on a steep hillside fenced to keep out roaming cattle. Privacy is excellent, views outstanding, and each individually named site unique (reservations are for specific sites). Reserve well in advance for summer weekends—the trail camp is often full. Outside of these times, space is usually available. Note that residents of Alameda and Contra Costa counties can make reservations beginning November 1 for the entire following year. *Fires, alcohol, dogs, and bicycles are prohibited.*

Site 1 (Sycamore), capacity 5, shades beneath sycamores near the top of the hill. Site 2 (Stars Rest), capacity 30, the largest site, is on top of the hill and has great views but limited shade. Site 3 (Hawks Rest), capacity 5, is small and shady with sweet rock outcrops and views. It's also closest to water, but has only one good tent site. Site 4 (Eagles

❾ Sunol Regional Wilderness: Sunol Backpack Camp Loop

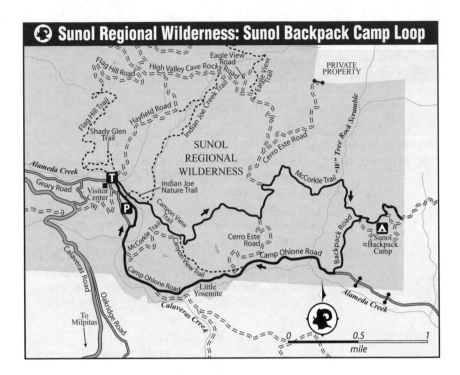

Eyrie), capacity 10, has limited shade and spectacular views and is close to water. Site 5 (Sky Camp), capacity 5, is very isolated and shady beneath blue oaks and has epic views. Site 6 (Cathedral Camp), capacity 10, is very shady near the bottom of the hill, has no views, and is far from water. Site 7 (Oak View), capacity 5, is very isolated near the bottom of the hill and has some shade beneath twisting blue oaks. It has good views but no picnic table, and is the farthest from water.

Getting There

Take Highway 680 east of Fremont to the Calaveras Road exit and proceed south on Calaveras Road for 4.3 miles to Geary Road. Turn left on Geary Road, reaching the visitor center parking lot and trailhead in 1.9 miles. There is a parking fee of $5.

Hiking It

The trail passes through numerous gates; leave them as you find them. Fill up at the trailhead before you start—there is no more water between here and Sunol Backpack Camp.

Begin the adventure across Geary Road at the wooden bridge over Alameda Creek. The largest watershed in the East Bay, Alameda Creek drains more than 700 square miles and is lined with the mottled, smooth gray trunks and twisting branches of California sycamores. These distinctive trees appear throughout Sunol in damp stream gullies, providing excellent shade. With their broad leaves, sycamores can lose up to 50 gallons of water per day and grow only where such large volumes of water are available. Also keep an eye out for poison oak and stinging nettle, ubiquitous and unfriendly companions on this hike.

Wildflowers are extraordinary from March through May, and you may see dozens of different species along the trail, including lupine, fiddlenecks, California poppies, western hound's tongue, brodiaea, baby blue eyes, witch hazel, shooting stars, buttercups, scarlet pimpernel, Chinese houses, and California gilia. The Sunol Visitor Center provides displays and handouts on the common flora and fauna encountered in the area.

Across the bridge, bear right on the wide path and continue straight on Canyon View Trail as it passes junctions on the left for Hayfield Road (0.1/410'), Indian Joe Nature Trail (0.2/410'), and Indian Joe Creek Trail (0.3/410'). Canyon View Trail soon climbs away from the creek and into a drier environment populated primarily by blue oaks, the most drought-tolerant of all oaks. Easily recognized, its leaves are shallowly lobed with smooth margins. After passing though one of numerous cattle gates to come, Canyon View Trail reaches a four-way intersection with McCorkle Trail (0.8/700'). Go left on McCorkle Trail. Cows are still permitted to graze throughout Sunol and are commonly seen in this area.

The narrower trail climbs steeply and steadily up the ridgeline before turning east to traverse through chaparral. The low-lying and shrubby chaparral community flourishes in arid environments

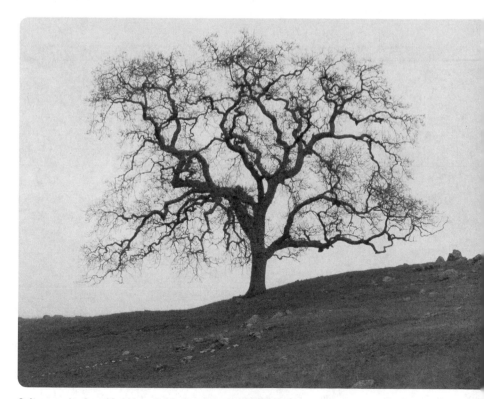

Oaks, grassland, and boulders define Sunol Regional Wilderness.

and appears throughout the hike. Common members include coyote brush, toyon, sticky monkeyflower, bracken fern, coffee berry, and plenty of poison oak. Valley oak, another frequent tree on this hike, also begins to appear along this section, identified by its 2- to 4-inch deeply lobed leaves. After passing beneath some huge coast live oaks, the trail reaches the junction with wide Cerro Este Road (1.7/1,180'). Bear left on Cerro Este Road, make the steady uphill climb to the next junction with McCorkle Trail (2.1/1,430'), and bear right on single-track McCorkle Trail.

Traversing steadily across open slopes, the trail offers outstanding views of Mission Peak to the west, and to the south the Calaveras Reservoir, the upper Alameda Creek watershed, and more distant peaks of the Diablo Range.

After making a switchbacking drop into a steep drainage, you continue the traverse to reach the junction with Backpack Road (3.4/1,150') and the gated edge of Sunol Backpack Camp.

After passing through the gate, the trail climbs steeply up the hillside. An almost indiscernible use path splits right just past the gate and lead to Sites 6–7. About halfway up the hillside, the main trail makes an unsigned fork. Bear right to reach Sites 3–5, or continue straight ahead to find Sites 1–2 near the top of the hill. The one water source is located right above Site 3. Interesting serpentine outcrops protrude from the hillside here, easily identified by the waxy green color found on unweathered surfaces.

To return to the trailhead, follow wide Backpack Road as it steadily de-

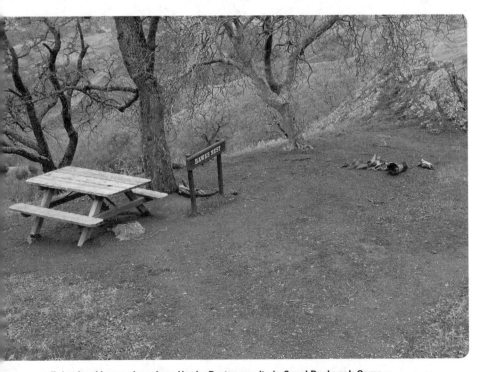

Enjoy hawk's-eye views from Hawks Rest campsite in Sunol Backpack Camp.

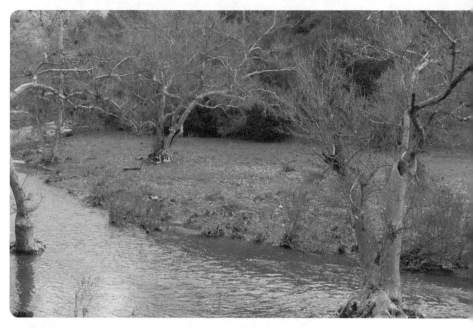

Sycamores line Alameda Creek.

scends to Camp Ohlone Road (4.0/800'), where you turn right to begin your tour alongside nearby Alameda Creek. It's an easy cruise along this wide thoroughfare to Little Yosemite (4.5/450'). With a rushing river coursing through a small gorge over boulders blue and green, Little Yosemite is a pretty sight. From here, continue on level Camp Ohlone Road to rejoin the park road at the upper parking lot (5.5/420'). Watch for gray pine, California buckeye, and the reappearance of coast live oak and California bay along this final section. Walk the road to return to the visitor center (5.9/410').

Giving Back

The **Regional Parks Foundation** supports and funds the acquisition, development, and stewardship of parklands in the East Bay Regional Park District through private contributions. Contact the foundation or learn more about their mission at (510) 544-2200 or **www.regionalparksfoundation.org**.

Anyone interested in volunteering for Sunol Regional Wilderness—or any other unit of the **East Bay Regional Park District**—can contact the district's volunteer coordinator for more information at (510) 544-2515 or volunteers@ebparks.org.

Alameda Creek Alliance is a community watershed group dedicated to preserving and restoring the natural ecosystems of the Alameda Creek drainage basin. Contact the alliance or learn more at (510) 499-9185 or **www.alamedacreek.org**.

22 Del Valle Regional Park:
MURIETTA FALLS LOOP

RATINGS	Scenery **7** Difficulty **8** Solitude **8**
ROUND-TRIP DISTANCE	4.2 miles to Boyd Camp 14.0 miles to Stewart's Camp
ELEVATION GAIN/LOSS	+1,600'/–1,600' to Boyd Camp +3,800'/–3,800' to Stewart's Camp
OPTIONAL MAPS	*Ohlone Wilderness Regional Trail Permit and Map* and *Del Valle Regional Park Map*, both by the East Bay Regional Park District
BEST TIMES	February through May
AGENCY	Del Valle Regional Park, (925) 373-0432, **www.ebparks.org/parks/ del_valle**. Park visitor center is open daily 10 a.m.–5:30 p.m. Memorial Day through Labor Day. Ohlone Regional Wilderness, (510) 544-3246, **www.ebparks.org/parks/ohlone**.
PERMIT	Trail camp permits ($5 per person, plus a one-time $8 reservation fee) can be reserved for the entire calendar year beginning February 1. Call 888-EBPARKS (327-2757), 8:30 a.m.–4 p.m. Monday–Friday. Campers can make last-minute arrangements at the park if space is available. The required *Ohlone Wilderness Regional Trail Permit and Map* ($2) is available at Del Valle or through the reservation office.

Highlights
Climb into the wilds of the East Bay Regional Park District to discover a wispy waterfall high in the mountainous hills of the Diablo Range. Beautiful oaks, prolific wildflowers, and far-reaching views provide accompaniment along this intense calf-burning hike.

Hike Overview
This journey ascends into the heart of Ohlone Regional Wilderness from Del Valle Regional Park, a strenuous hike that rapidly gains more than 3,000 feet to reach the upper elevations of the Diablo Range. En route, near the midpoint of the climb, you reach Boyd Camp, a pleasant overnight destination in itself or an excellent base camp for exploring the higher reaches. The latter

half of the ascent climbs a steep section aptly named the "Big Burn" to reach a broad and pleasant vale sheltering Stewart's Camp and thin Murietta Falls.

Spring, when wildflowers peak and temperatures are optimal, is the ideal time to visit. Flowers peak and trees leaf out at lower elevations the last week of March and first week of April; at higher elevations full spring glory arrives in mid- to late April. Summer and fall are also possibilities, though days can be oppressively hot, especially on unshaded sections of trail.

Trail Camps
Two trail camps are available: Boyd Camp and Stewart's Camp. **Boyd Camp** hides at an elevation of 2,200 feet on moderately forested slopes of blue oak,

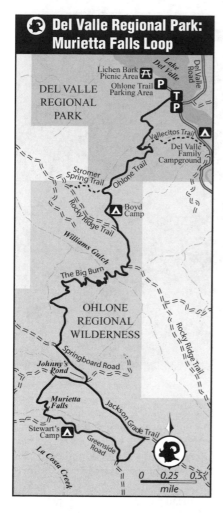

⊘ Del Valle Regional Park: Murietta Falls Loop

DEL VALLE REGIONAL PARK

Lichen Bark Picnic Area
Ohlone Trail Parking Area

Lake Del Valle
Del Valle Road

Vallecitos Trail
Del Valle Family Campground

Stromer Spring Trail
Ohlone Trail

Boyd Camp

Rocky Ridge Trail

Williams Gulch

The Big Burn

OHLONE REGIONAL WILDERNESS

Rocky Ridge Trail

Springboard Road

Johnny's Pond

Murietta Falls

Jackson Grade Trail

Stewart's Camp

Greenside Road

La Costa Creek

0   0.25   0.5
mile

a small grassy clearing with less shade but much more space.

Stewart's Camp, at 3,160 feet, offers only one site, and is located on the shady edge of a vast open valley populated almost exclusively by massive black oaks. The small site is located near water and an outhouse, and is surrounded by a denser forest of live oaks, bay, and buckeyes. Space is limited, but up to 24 people are permitted to camp in the site.

Reservations are for specific sites. *Fires, alcohol, dogs, and bicycles are prohibited.* Residents of Alameda and Contra Costa counties can make reservations beginning November 1 for the entire following year.

Getting There

Take the North Livermore Avenue exit from Interstate 580. Head south and proceed through town (North Livermore Avenue becomes South Livermore Avenue). About 1.5 miles outside town, turn right at Mines Road, go about 3.5 miles, and continue straight on Del Valle Road as Mines Road turns left. The park entrance is about 3.5 miles ahead. Past the entrance station continue on Del Valle Road for 0.8 mile, cross the bridge, and turn right to the Lichen Bark Picnic Area and Ohlone Trail Parking Area.

Hiking It

black oak, and gray pine. The camp is only 2 miles from the trailhead, but access requires a sustained and heart-pumping climb of 1,300 vertical feet, which limits the number of visitors. There are two sites, both nicely removed from the trail and, unfortunately, the water; the only water source is a year-round spring located almost a half mile and 300 vertical feet below camp. Site 1 is smaller and situated beneath shady blue oaks. Site 2 is on the edge of

This route follows the eastern portion of the Ohlone Trail, a long-distance hiking trail that runs from Mission Peak in Fremont to Del Valle Reservoir in Livermore. The Ohlone Trail is a route comprised of many different trails. Many junctions—but not all—will be posted and indicate the correct direction for the Ohlone Trail. Most are numbered to correspond with the Ohlone Trail permit and map. The trail

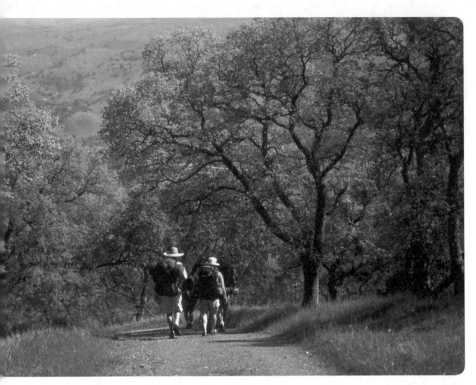

Down, down, down to Del Valle

passes through numerous gates—leave them as you find them.

From Lichen Bark Picnic Area (0.0/750'), begin on the Ohlone Trail as it makes a steadily ascending traverse on Sailor Camp Trail to reach a junction on the left with Vallecitos Trail (0.9/1,190'), which leads directly to the Del Valle Family Campground. Record your visit in the logbook at the adjacent Ohlone Trail sign-in panel; an Ohlone Trail permit is required past this point.

Continue straight on the Ohlone Trail to quickly begin a direct, calf-burning ascent on a wide path through a mixed environment of blue and coast live oaks, gray pines, and thick chaparral. Manzanita, coyote brush, coffee berry, and toyon predominate in the low-lying brush; coast live oaks intermittently join their blue oak brethren overhead. Coast live oaks peter out as you pass through a gate, cross into Ohlone Regional Wilderness, and reach Stromer Spring Trail (1.7/1,940'); water is available a short distance down the path to your right. A final straight-line ascent brings you to Boyd Camp (2.1/2,240').

Past Boyd Camp, the trail continues its steep climb, curving left to complete the final leg of the hike's initial ascent and reach Rocky Ridge Trail

(2.3/2,380'). The route now gently descends through open fields of blue oak with intermittent views of Mt. Diablo, then begins a steep switchbacking descent into Williams Gulch. The trail narrows as it drops to reach an ephemeral creek at the bottom (2.8/1,890'), flowing beneath water-loving sycamores and alders.

Now the "Big Burn" begins. The trail narrows to single-track and climbs a section of seemingly endless switchbacks to gain 1,400 feet of elevation in only 1.7 miles. On this north-facing slope, shaded from sun's rays, the vegetation is dense, blocks the view, and encroaches on the trail in many places. Wild cucumber, maidenhair ferns, gooseberry, black oaks, bay trees, and thick poison oak are common on this shady section.

Ultimately you reach the junction with Springboard Road (5/3,300'), where the gradient finally eases. Bear left to remain on the Ohlone Trail (here Jackson Grade Trail), which now resumes its broad character. Winding through open oak-studded terrain, you enjoy outstanding views of San Francisco and Sutro Tower, the East Bay Hills, Mission Peak to the southwest, and Lake Del Valle to the north.

You next encounter Johnny's Pond (5.0/3,350') at a four-way intersection with Springboard Road. Here, at the highest point of your heart-pounding journey, the time has come to stop and relax. Look north and west for distant views of Mt. Tamalpais, the Golden Gate, and Mt. Diablo. Immediately behind you, the upper watershed of La Costa Creek is punctuated by gigantic blue and black oaks in open fields flush with wildflowers. The steep, inviting landscape is easy to explore in all directions. Stewart's Camp sits in the bottom of the valley on the west side of La Costa Creek.

To continue to Murietta Falls and Stewart's Camp, leave the Ohlone Trail and bear right on Springboard Road to quickly reach the junction with Greenside Trail (5.3/3,280'). Turn left to descend Greenside Trail, dropping steeply into the headwaters of La Costa Creek to reach the trickling waterway at valley bottom (5.8/3,000'). Murietta Falls is nearby and can be reached by following the obvious use paths downstream. Dropping 60 feet in a thin rivulet on a rocky cliff face, the waterfall is seldom more than a thin trickle. More interesting are the rocky outcrops and exciting scramble required to access the falls.

If Stewart's Camp is your final destination, proceed across the creek and briefly climb, bearing left at the junction with Greenside Trail (5.9/3,070'). From here, follow Greenside Trail as it traverses past shadier slopes of bay, live oak, and buckeye to reach the camp's outhouse, water source, and campsite (6.3/3,160'). Return the way you came.

Giving Back

The **Regional Parks Foundation** supports and funds the acquisition, development, and stewardship of parklands in the East Bay Regional Park District through private contributions. Contact the foundation or learn more at (510) 544-2200 or **www.regionalparks foundation.org.**

Anyone interested in volunteering for parks along the Ohlone Trail—or any other unit of the **East Bay Regional Park District**—can contact the district's volunteer coordinator for more information at (510) 544-2515 or volunteers @ebparks.org.

23 The Ohlone Trail

RATINGS	Scenery **10** Difficulty **8** Solitude **9**
ONE-WAY DISTANCE	28.2 miles
ELEVATION GAIN/LOSS	+8,500'/–8,150'
OPTIONAL MAPS	*Ohlone Wilderness Regional Trail Permit and Map* and *Mission Peak Regional Preserve, Sunol Regional Wilderness,* and *Del Valle Regional Park* maps, all by the East Bay Regional Park District
BEST TIMES	Spring and fall
AGENCY	Mission Peak Regional Preserve, (510) 544-3246, **www.ebparks.org/ parks/mission**; Sunol Regional Wilderness, (510) 544-3249, **www. ebparks.org/parks/sunol**; Ohlone Regional Wilderness, (510) 544-3246, **www.ebparks.org/parks/ohlone**; Del Valle Regional Park, (925) 373-0432, **www.ebparks.org/parks/del_valle**; East Bay Regional Park District, 888-EBPARKS, **www.ebparks.org**.
PERMIT	The *Ohlone Wilderness Regional Trail Permit and Map* ($2) is required, which you can purchase at Sunol, Del Valle, or through the EBRPD reservations office. Trail camp reservations ($5 per person, plus a one-time $8 reservation fee) can be made for the entire calendar year beginning February 1. Call 888-EBPARKS (327-2757), 8:30 a.m.–4 p.m. Monday–Friday. Reservations are recommended, though last-minute arrangements can be made at Sunol and Del Valle if space is available.

Highlights

Stretching 28 miles through the most remote land in the East Bay Regional Park District, the Ohlone Trail is a point-to-point journey remarkable for its isolation, beauty, and strenuous hiking. The adventure connects Mission Peak Regional Preserve and Sunol Regional Wilderness to Del Valle Regional Park via Ohlone Regional Wilderness, a hidden, high-elevation wonderland accessible only by trail. The proximity of such a lightly traveled hike to civilization is exceptional.

Hike Overview

Strenuous and constant elevation change across hilly terrain defines the entire measure of the Ohlone Trail. A minimum of three days is recommended to complete it; four leisurely days is

delightful. A car shuttle or prearranged pick-up is required at trail's end. While hiking the entire trail in two days is possible, it allows little time for relaxation and enjoyment. Better two-day trips are possible by hiking out-and-back to the closest trail camps from the respective trailheads. Note also that you can skip the Mission Peak portion (and its 8.6 miles and 2,000 feet of elevation change) by starting the hike instead from Sunol Regional Wilderness, the only other access point.

The Ohlone Trail can be completed in either direction; the trip is described from west to east, Mission Peak to Del Valle, in the direction of more gradual elevation gain (beginning at Del Valle necessitates a 2,500-foot climb with full packs in the first 5 miles, a burning introduction to the adventure). The

The Ohlone Trail

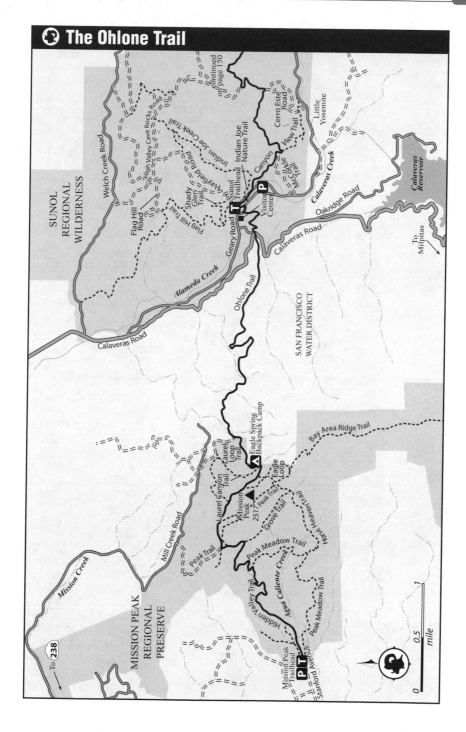

continued off page 150

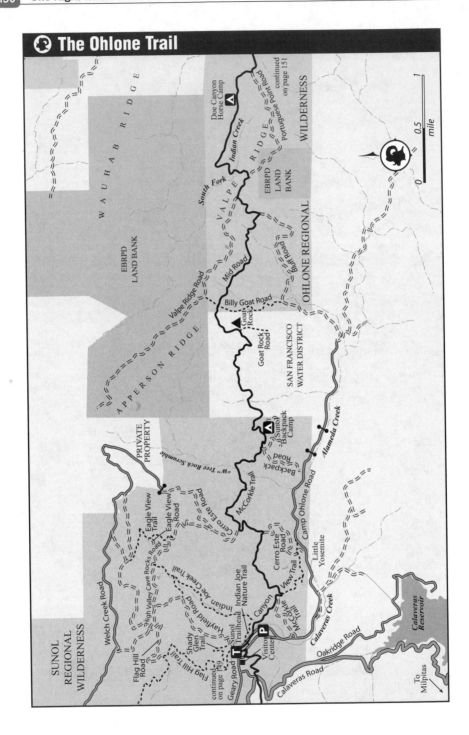

The Ohlone Trail

◎ The Ohlone Trail

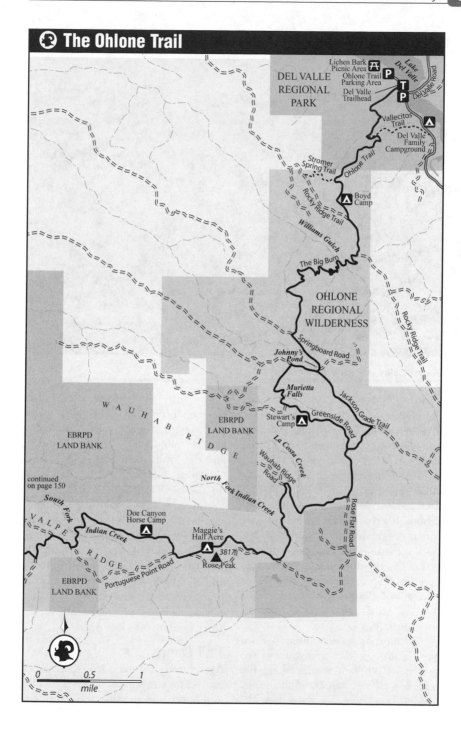

Lichen Bark 🏕 🅿
Picnic Area
Ohlone Trail 🅿
Parking Area
DEL VALLE 🅿 🚾
REGIONAL Del Valle 🚾
PARK Del Valle
Trailhead

Lake
Del Valle

Del Valle Road

Vallecitos
Trail 🔺
Del Valle
Family
Campground

Stromer
Spring Trail

Ohlone Trail

Rocky Ridge Trail

🔺 Boyd
Camp

Williams Gulch

The Big Burn

**OHLONE
REGIONAL
WILDERNESS**

Rocky Ridge Trail

Springboard Road

*Johnny's
Pond*

*Murietta
Falls*

Jackson Grade Trail

Stewart's 🔺 *Greenside Road*
Camp

W A U H A B   EBRPD
LAND BANK

R I D G E   *La Costa Creek*

EBRPD
LAND BANK

*Wauhab Ridge
Road*

continued
on page 150

North *Fork Indian Creek*

Rose Flat Road

South
Fork

Doe Canyon
Horse Camp
🔺

Maggie's
Half Acre
🔺

V A L P E

Indian Creek

R I D G E   3817'
▲
Rose Peak

EBRPD
LAND BANK

Portuguese Point Road

0   0.5   1
mile

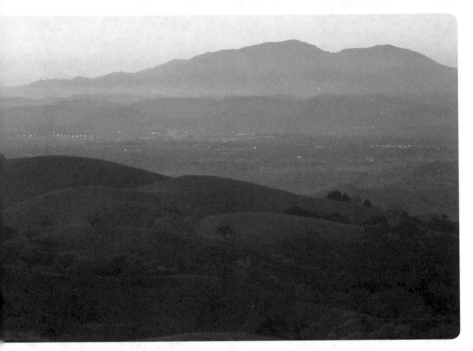

Mount Diablo looms north of Del Valle.

required *Ohlone Wilderness Regional Trail Permit and Map* provides excellent and detailed information about the hike.

The hills are lofty for the Bay Area—more than 7 miles of trail travel above 3,000 feet, making weather conditions highly variable. Summer sun can be oppressive on miles of unshaded trail, while the cold heights—and even possibility of snow—make winter less appealing. Spring is primetime for this hike as wildflowers explode in one of the Bay Area's most dazzling and diverse displays.

Wildflowers are extraordinary from March through May, and you may see dozens of different species along the trail, including lupine, fiddlenecks, California poppies, western hound's tongue, brodiaea, baby blue eyes, witch hazel, shooting stars, buttercups, scarlet pimpernel, Chinese houses, and California gilia. The Sunol Visitor Center provides displays and handouts on the common flora and fauna encountered in the area. Note that spring reaches the higher elevations on this hike several weeks later than at lower elevations. Wildflowers peak and trees leaf out below 1,000 feet in Sunol and Del Valle during the last week of March and first week of April; higher elevations don't experience full spring glory until mid- to late April.

Trail Camps

Backcountry camping is limited to six trail camps, each of which provides outhouses and potable water (except in the driest of conditions). From west to east they are Eagle Spring Backpack Camp, Sunol Backpack Camp, Doe Canyon Horse Camp, Maggie's Half Acre, Stewart's Camp, and Boyd Camp. Each is described in detail below. Reservations are for specific sites—the information below will help you request an ideal location.

Despite the heat, summer weekends are the busiest and many trail camps are full. Outside of these times, space is usually available. Residents of Alameda and Contra Costa counties can make reservations early, beginning November 1 for the entire following year. *Fires, alcohol, dogs, and bicycles are prohibited on the Ohlone Trail.*

For a leisurely four-day trip, the recommended camping areas in order are Eagle Spring (a short first day, providing ample time to shuttle vehicles), Sunol Backpack Camp, and either Stewart's Camp (making Day 3 the longest and most strenuous) or Maggie's Half Acre (Day 4 is the strenuous one). For those aiming to complete the hike in 3 days, aim for Sunol Backpack Camp and either Stewart's Camp or Maggie's Half Acre, regardless of whether you start from the Sunol or the Mission Peak Trailhead.

Eagle Spring Backpack Camp is situated on the east side of Mission Peak, perched just below the summit at 2,200 feet. Four sites are available. Three are exposed with no shade or wind protection, the fourth sits beneath the shady boughs of a large bay tree. Each has its own picnic table. The camp is fenced to keep out the many roving bovines; a water pump and outhouse are available. Excellent views look east into the oak-studded wilds of the Diablo Range.

Sunol Backpack Camp offers seven sites scattered across 500 vertical feet on a steep hillside fenced to keep out roaming cattle. Privacy is excellent, views outstanding, and each individually named site unique. Site 1 (Sycamore), capacity 5, shades beneath sycamores near the top of the hill. Site 2 (Stars Rest), capacity 30, the largest site, is on top of the hill, and has great views but limited shade except for the picnic table. Site 3 (Hawks Rest), capacity 5, is small and shady with sweet rock outcrops and views. It's also closest to water, but only has one good tent site. Site 4 (Eagles Eyrie), capacity 10, has limited shade and spectacular views and is close to water. Site 5 (Sky Camp), capacity 5, is very isolated and shady beneath blue oaks and has epic views. Site 6 (Cathedral Camp), capacity 10, is very shady near the bottom of the hill, has no views, and is far from water. Site 7 (Oak View), capacity 5, is very isolated near the bottom of the hill and has some shade beneath twisting blue oaks. It has good views but no picnic table, and is the farthest from water.

Doe Canyon Horse Camp provides two sites designed for use by equestrian groups, but backpackers are permitted to camp here if space is available. The trail camp is located at an elevation of 3,300 feet and consists of two large clearings situated amid low-lying brush. An outhouse, water, hitching posts, and limited views are nearby.

Maggie's Half Acre provides three sites at an elevation of 3,480 feet on the upper flanks of Rose Peak (3,817'), making this the highest designated campsite in the Bay Area. Despite its lofty location, views are obscured by a dense surrounding forest of live oaks, gray pine, bay, and some very gnarly black oaks. Sites 1 and 3 are positioned away from the trail in shady worlds beneath ancient oaks and have a capacity of 4–6 people. Site 2 is larger, located by the path and water, and accommodates up to 14 people. City lights peek through the shady canopy at night.

Stewart's Camp, at 3,160 feet, offers only one site and is located on the shady edge of a vast open valley populated almost exclusively by massive black oaks. The small site is located near the water and outhouse, and is surrounded by a denser forest of live oaks, bay, and buckeyes. Space is limited, but up to 24 people are permitted to camp in the site.

Boyd Camp hides at an elevation of 2,200 feet on moderately forested slopes of blue oak, black oak, and gray pine. The camp is only 2 miles from the Del Valle Trailhead, but access requires a heart-pumping climb of 1,300 vertical feet, which limits the number of visitors. There are two sites, both nicely removed from the trail and, unfortunately, the water; the only source is a year-round spring located almost a half mile and 300 vertical feet below camp. Site 1 is smaller and beneath shady blue oaks adjacent to an unusually nice buckeye tree. Site 2 is on the edge of a small grassy clearing with less shade but much more space.

Getting There

To reach the Mission Peak Trailhead, take I-680 to Fremont. From northbound I-680, take the Mission Boulevard exit, and proceed straight on Mission Boulevard 0.7 mile. Turn right on Stanford Avenue and proceed 0.6 mile to the parking lot and trailhead. From southbound I-680, take the exit for Mission Boulevard and Highway 238, turn left on Mission Boulevard, go 2.8 miles, turn left on Stanford Avenue, and proceed as above. Public transportation is possible—AC Transit #217 runs from the Fremont BART Station to Stanford Avenue and Mission Bou-

levard. Check schedules and service at (510) 817-1717 or **www.actransit.org.**

To reach the Sunol Trailhead, take I-680 east of Fremont to the Calaveras Road exit, and proceed south on Calaveras Road for 4.3 miles to Geary Road. Turn left on Geary Road, reaching the entrance kiosk in 1.8 miles. The trailhead is located across Geary Road from the Ohlone Trail sign-in panel, approximately 100 yards past the visitor center.

To reach the Del Valle Trailhead, take the North Livermore Avenue exit from I-580. Head south and proceed through town (North Livermore Avenue becomes South Livermore Avenue). About 1.5 miles outside town, turn right at Mines Road, go about 3.5 miles, and continue straight on Del Valle Road as Mines Road turns left. The park entrance is about 3.5 miles ahead. Past the entrance station continue on Del Valle Road for 0.8 mile, cross the bridge, and turn right to the Lichen Bark Picnic Area and Ohlone Trail Parking Area.

To reach the Sunol Trailhead from the Del Valle Trailhead, return to central Livermore and turn left onto 1st Street. Proceed 0.6 mile on 1st Street to Holmes Road and turn left. In 2 miles, bear right on the combination Vallecitos Road and Highway 84 and continue for another 6.5 miles to I-680. Go underneath the freeway, turn left on Paloma Road, pass back beneath 680, and go straight at the next stop onto Calaveras Road. Continue as above.

Hiking It

The Ohlone Trail is a route comprised of many different trails. Many junctions—but not all—will be posted and indicate the correct direction for the Ohlone Trail. Most are numbered to correspond with the Ohlone Trail per-

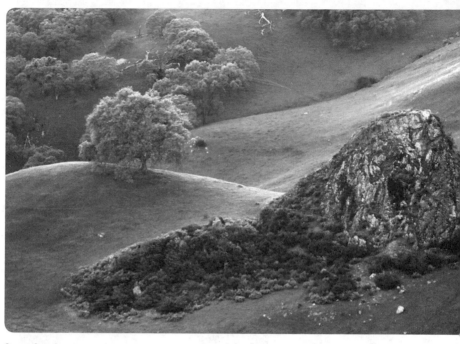

Sweet Sunol

mit and map. The trail passes through numerous gates—leave them as you find them. Water sources are generally scarce, with the only sure supplies available at the trail camps. Fill up at the trailhead before you start.

MISSION PEAK TO SUNOL Your journey begins at the gate (0.0/410') on a wide fire road. The entire western flank of Mission Peak (2,517') rises before you, laced by the watershed of Agua Caliente Creek. Cattle browse the grassy hillsides. Ohlone Trail signpost 1 (OT 1) quickly appears, the first of many numbered postings listed on the *Ohlone Wilderness Regional Trail Permit and Map*.

Continue straight as Peak Meadow Trail forks to the right (0.2/470'). Your wide path curves left toward more open views, passing a copse of coast live oak on the right. Look for buckeye and sycamore trees in the small nearby creek gully. The trail bears right to cross this small drainage, then curves and briefly parallels Agua Caliente Creek before crossing a cattle guard to enter the fenced-off world of cattle country. Looking behind you to the west, Coyote Hills dimple the horizon beyond Fremont.

Now steadily climbing, you curve upward to attain a discernible ridgeline. As you crest 1,000 feet in elevation, the trail briefly eases to pass the first of several benches overlooking the South Bay and the East of the Bay beyond. The sustained ascent next passes Peak Meadow Trail on the right (1.5/1,490') and reaches a cattle guard below the rocky ramparts of the summit massif.

Large sandstone (graywacke) boulders rest on the slopes, a lone coast live oak holds a tenuous foothold below, and a park residence is visible ahead in the distance across the meadow.

Bear left at the next junction with Grove Trail (2.2/1,810') to quickly reach another junction (2.4/1,990')—go right on the rougher and more rutted road. At signpost 4 (2.5/2,060'), views north open up toward Mount Diablo

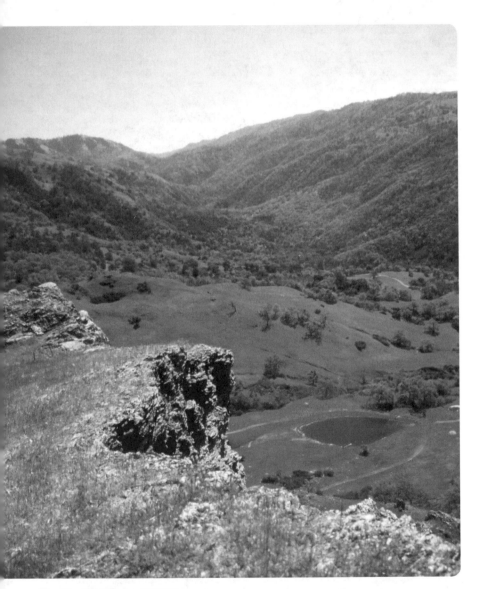

The Alameda Creek watershed

and the East Bay Hills as you round the shoulder of Mission Peak. Continuing right on Eagle Trail, you soon encounter a junction with Peak Trail (2.7/2,130') and attain your first views east into the hills of Sunol Regional Wilderness and Ohlone Regional Wilderness—your continuing route. Remain on Eagle Trail as it traverses past signpost 6 (2.9/2,050') to reach signpost 7 and the trail camp (3.0/2,200').

The summit and its sweeping views are within easy striking distance from camp; fully survey it on a 1.7-mile loop via Eagle and Peak trails (elevation gain and loss of +550'/-550'). The loop can be completed in either direction; clockwise is recommended. A unique pipe viewer on the summit identifies distant landmarks; you can see San Francisco, Mount Tamalpais, the East Bay, and the entire South Bay.

The Ohlone Trail descends east past the trail camp on a wide path, quickly dropping into a shady creek corridor of coast live oaks, bay trees, and intermittent black oaks. The route crosses the stream and hits a junction for Laurel Canyon Trail on the left (3.2/2,050'). Continue straight on the Ohlone Trail into open hillsides, cruising past extensive meadows of cows. You encounter the far end of single-track Laurel Loop Trail (3.6/1,900') on the left before immediately reaching a large gate and sign marking the watershed boundary.

At this point you leave the East Bay Regional Park District and begin traveling by trail easement across San Francisco Water District land—respect this arrangement and stay on the trail in the miles ahead. Cross the gate and bear right, soon curving across a shady stream gulch flush with poison oak and beginning a downhill traverse past coast live oak, bay trees, and some large black oaks.

Intermittent Ohlone Trail signs lead you on as you continue straight at a junction by a break in barbed wire, next pass through an open gate, and then reenter the woods again. Views open up east of Sunol Regional Wilderness as the wide road traverses a cow-filled landscape. A keen eye can pick out the Sunol Backpack Camp immediately beyond a prominent rock outcrop due east.

The route makes a broad switchback left and winds past some nice valley and blue oaks. You cross a private road (5.2/1,570'), then make a steadier descent among coast live oak, madrone, and black oak. Chaparral species appear in some spots, including toyon, coffee berry, honey suckle, coyote brush, and lots of poison oak. The descent soon steepens and drops along a ridgeline among thick and diverse oak trees.

Paved Calaveras Road becomes visible below and is soon met as the trail reaches a gate alongside the pavement (6.5/870'). Cross the road to enter Sunol Regional Wilderness, and bear left on a thin single-track trail. You briefly travel below and parallel to the road, then curve away to the right and descend a small ridgeline. The route switchbacks left, drops gently through pleasant blue oak woodlands, and then turns right to pass through a fence. The posted trail soon cruises level; stay left at the fork and make a final switchback to reach the Ohlone Trail sign-in board and parking area (8.7/410').

SUNOL VISITOR CENTER TO SUNOL BACKPACK CAMP Register at the Ohlone Trail sign-in board and begin the adventure at the wooden bridge over Alameda Creek. Alameda Creek is the largest watershed in the East Bay, draining more than 700 square miles, and its deep valleys are your regular companions during the first half of the trip. The mottled, smooth gray trunks and twisting branches of California sycamores line the creek and appear throughout the Ohlone Trail in damp stream gullies, providing excellent shade. With their broad leaves, sycamore trees can lose up to 50 gallons of water per day and grow only where such large volumes of water are available. Also keep an eye out for poison oak and stinging nettle, ubiquitous and unfriendly companions on this hike.

Across the bridge, bear right on the wide path and continue straight on Canyon View Trail as it passes junctions on the left for Hayfield Road (8.8/410'), Indian Joe Nature Trail (8.9/410'), and Indian Joe Creek Trail (9.0/410'). Canyon View Trail soon climbs away from the creek and into a drier environment populated primarily by blue oaks, the most drought-tolerant of all oaks. Easily recognized, its leaves are shallowly lobed with smooth margins. After passing though one of numerous cattle gates to come, Canyon View Trail reaches a four-way intersection with McCorkle Trail (9.5/700'). Go left on McCorkle Trail. Cows are still permitted to graze along much of the Ohlone Trail and are commonly seen in this area.

The now overgrown trail climbs steadily up the ridgeline before turning east to traverse through chaparral. The low-lying and shrubby chaparral community flourishes in arid environments and appears throughout the hike. Common members include coyote brush, toyon, sticky monkeyflower, bracken fern, coffee berry, and plenty of poison oak. Valley oak, another frequent tree on this hike, also begins to appear along this section, identified by its 2- to 4-inch deeply lobed leaves. After passing beneath some huge coast live oaks, the trail then reaches the junction with

wide Cerro Este Road (10.4/1,180'). Bear left on Cerro Este Road, make the steady uphill climb to the next junction with McCorkle Trail (10.8/1,430'), and bear right on single-track McCorkle Trail. Traversing steadily across open slopes, the trail offers outstanding views of Mission Peak to the west, and to the south the Calaveras Reservoir, the upper Alameda Creek watershed, and more distant peaks of the Diablo Range. After making a switchbacking drop into a steep ravine known as the "W" Tree Rock Scramble, the trail continues its traverse to reach the junction with Backpack Road (12.1/1,150') and the gated edge of Sunol Backpack Camp.

After passing through the gate, the trail climbs steeply up the hillside. An almost indiscernible use path splits right just past the gate and lead to Sites 6–7. About halfway up the hillside, the main trail makes an unsigned fork. Bear right to reach Sites 3–5, or continue straight ahead to find Sites 1–2 near the top of the hill. The one water source is located right above Site 3. Interesting serpentine outcrops protrude from the hillside here, easily identified by the waxy green color found on unweathered surfaces.

SUNOL BACKPACK CAMP TO STEWART'S CAMP After a delightful night, the next day begins with a climb to the top of the hill where a gate marks the edge of Sunol Regional Wilderness. For the next 2 miles the trail passes through land leased from the San Francisco Water District—*stay on the trail during this section.* Undulating through open serpentine grasslands dotted with rock outcrops and fabulous spring wildflower displays, the open trail provides far-reaching views as it traverses the upper slopes of the Alameda Creek drainage. The trail winds above Goat

Rock, a distinctive promontory composed of erosion-resistant red chert, and then turns uphill. Bear left at the first unposted junction with Goat Rock Road (5.3/2,170') and right at the second junction (14.2/2,320') to continue westward on Mid Road.

Shortly thereafter you pass through another gate and enter Ohlone Regional Wilderness just before reaching the four-way junction with Billy Goat Road (14.5/2,390'). The route continues straight on Mid Road and begins a rising traverse slowly toward the ridgeline above. The cities of the South Bay begin to appear in the southern distance, while intermittent views of distant South San Francisco can be spotted to the northwest. The trail turns left at the junction with Bluff Road (15.8/2,650'), and then climbs to the ridgeline and junction with Valpe Ridge Road (16.1/2,840').

Go right on Valpe Ridge Road, through another gate, and proceed along the airy slopes. As the trail banks left at the junction with Portuguese Point Road (16.4/2,920'), it leaves the upper Alameda Creek watershed for the first time and drops into the headwaters of Indian Creek, a separate drainage that rejoins Alameda Creek near Interstate 680.

After crossing South Fork Indian Creek, the trail resumes its climb and soon passes above 3,000 feet for the first time. Views north begin to appear and the massif of Mt. Diablo (3,849') is easily spotted more than 25 miles distant. At this higher elevation, black oaks also begin to appear for the first time. A common denizen of higher elevations around the state, black oaks are relatively uncommon in the Bay Area and found only at higher

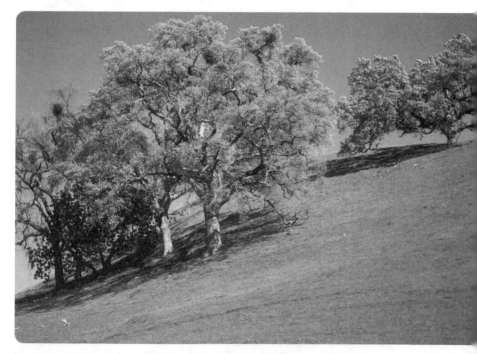

Beautiful oak trees shade the hillsides of Ohlone Regional Wilderness.

elevations in the Diablo Range and East of the Bay. They are easily identified by their large, lobed leaves, and leaf points ending in a pointy bristle. In spring their new leaves emerge a brilliant red before turning green. The wispy, multitrunked forms of gray pine become more common as well, and the evergreen leaves of live oaks start to appear. Thankfully, poison oak diminishes considerably at these higher elevations.

A short side trip 200 feet downhill at the junction for Doe Canyon Horse Camp (17.6/3,380') leads to the large clearing, water source, and outhouse by the campsites. Continuing, the trail reaches another junction with Portuguese Point Road (18.0/3,540') after passing through a gate held shut with a loop of barbed wire. Continue straight to quickly reach the spur trail on the left for the campsites at Maggie's Half Acre (18.2/3,590'), a quarter mile down the forested north slopes of Rose Peak.

While the trail to Maggie's Half Acre traverses around to rejoin the main trail 0.6 mile past the campsites, it bypasses the summit of Rose Peak (3,817'). A side trip you should not miss, Rose Peak is only 32 feet lower than Mt. Diablo, is the highest point on the hike, and offers extraordinary 360-degree views. On a good day, the vista stretches from San Francisco to the Sierra Nevada; its key landmarks are highlighted on the Ohlone Trail permit and map. A large plastic cylinder protects a summit register for

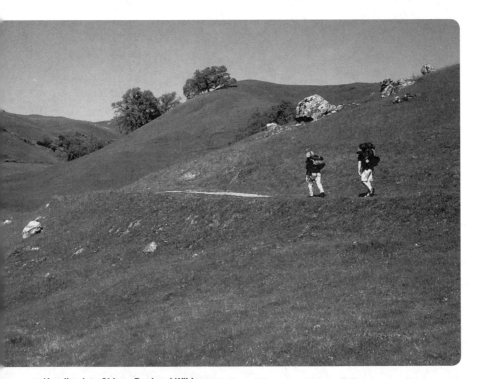

Heading into Ohlone Regional Wilderness

personal notes, contributions, and reflections. To reach Rose Peak, continue on the Ohlone Trail past the trail camp junction and make the short detour to the top from the main trail as it skirts just below the summit.

Continuing past Rose Peak, you pass the opposite junction for Maggie's Half Acre (18.9/3,590') and then briefly parallel the fenced park boundary where a private road splits right (19.2/3,590'). Curving left, the trail begins its northern journey to Del Valle after 10 miles of westward progression.

After plummeting more than 400 feet to cross shady North Fork Indian Creek, the trail then climbs the more open opposite slopes. Look down the Indian Creek drainage to spot the small, rounded forms of Coyote Hills, visible on the edge of the Bay, marking the location where Alameda Creek joins the Bay. After passing a junction for Wauhab Ridge Road (20.2/3,490') on the left, the route cuts back to attain the ridgetop and then dips down into the head of Box Canyon. Passing a small cattle pond, the trail climbs along the park boundary, turns left at the junction with Rose Flat Road (21.1/3,640'), and then gently undulates north to reach the junction with Greenside Trail ((21.6/3,490').

To reach Stewart's Camp from here, turn left and descend 0.6 mile on Greenside Trail to the outhouse, water source, and campsite. Those staying overnight here can rejoin the Ohlone Trail by continuing on Greenside Trail and bearing right on Springboard Road to reach Johnny's Pond.

STEWART'S CAMP TO DEL VALLE TRAILHEAD From the Greenside Trail junction, the Ohlone Trail continues straight across the open meadows of Shafer Flat to reach the junction with Jackson Grade Trail (22.0/3,460') and head left (northwest) along the ridgeline that hems in the beautiful valley of upper La Costa Creek. Gigantic blue and black oaks punctuate open fields flourishing with wildflowers and the steep, inviting landscape is easy to explore in all directions. Stewart's Camp (3,160') sits in the bottom of the valley on the west side of La Costa Creek.

Reaching Johnny's Pond at a four-way intersection with Springboard Road (22.7/3,350'), the time has come to stop and relax. With distant views reaching north to Mt. Tamalpais, the Golden Gate, and Mt. Diablo, plus a nearby waterfall to explore, this is no time to rush. Murietta Falls (2,990') is located along Greenside Trail, a half mile west of Stewart's Camp and a mile from Johnny's Pond via Springboard Road and Greenside Trail. Dropping 60 feet in a thin rivulet on a rocky cliff face, the waterfall is seldom more than a thin trickle. More interesting are the rocky outcrops and exciting scramble required to access the falls. To find Murietta Falls, follow the use paths downstream where Greenside Trail crosses La Costa Creek.

From Johnny's Pond, the Ohlone Trail continues straight on Jackson Grade Trail and offers ever vaster views of San Francisco and Sutro Tower, the East Bay hills, Mission Peak, and north to your final destination, Lake Del Valle. Enjoy these final high-elevation views, for once you turn right at the junction for the "Big Burn" (23.3/3,300'), the plummeting descent to trail's end begins.

Dropping immediately, the broad trail soon narrows to single-track, and poison oak once again rears its ugly leaves. On this north-facing slope, shaded from sun's rays, the vegetation is dense, blocks the view, and also encroaches on the trail in many places. Wild cucumber, maidenhair ferns, and gooseberry join bay, black oak, and thick poison oak on this shady section. Dropping endlessly on numerous switchbacks, the trail loses 1,400 feet of elevation in only 1.7 miles before finally reaching the bottom of Williams Gulch (25.0/1,890'). Here you pass beneath sycamores and alders while crossing the ephemeral creek. The trail gradually widens to become a broad path as it switchbacks steeply out of Williams Gulch and passes through open fields of blue oak with intermittent views north to Mt. Diablo. It reaches the Rocky Ridge Trail junction (25.7/2,380') at the end of the hike's final sustained climb.

Continuing straight, you resume the steep drop to quickly reach the outhouse and campsites of Boyd Camp (25.9/2,240') in a shrubbier forest of blue oak, gray pine, coyote brush, toyon, and coffee berry. From Boyd Camp the trail takes a direct, knee-jarring line straight down, passing the junction for water at Stromer Spring Trail (26.3/1,940') just before coast live oak reappears, and the trail passes through another gate. Manzanita appears for the first time on the hike, and coyote brush becomes increasingly common on the continuing descent.

Take the time to record your passing in the logbook where the trail reaches the Ohlone Trail sign-in panel by the junction with Vallecitos Trail (27.2/1,190'). Vallecitos Trail heads right down a creek gully toward the campground, while the Ohlone Trail continues straight on a steadily descending traverse to finally reach trail's end at Lichen Bark Picnic Area (28.2/750'). Good work!

Giving Back

The **Regional Parks Foundation** supports and funds the acquisition, development, and stewardship of parklands in the East Bay Regional Park District through private contributions. Contact the foundation or learn more at (510) 544-2200 or **www.regionalparks foundation.org.**

Anyone interested in volunteering for a park along the Ohlone Trail can contact the **East Bay Regional Park District**'s volunteer coordinator for more information at (510) 544-2515 or volunteers@ebparks.org.

Alameda Creek Alliance is a community watershed group dedicated to preserving and restoring the natural ecosystems of the Alameda Creek drainage basin. Contact the alliance or learn more at (510) 499-9185 or **www. alamedacreek.org.**

24 Henry W. Coe State Park:
THE WESTERN ZONE LOOP

RATINGS Scenery **7** Difficulty **7** Solitude **5**

ROUND-TRIP DISTANCE 12.1 miles

ELEVATION GAIN/LOSS +2,500'/–2,500'

RECOMMENDED MAP *Henry W. Coe State Park Trail and Camping Map* by the Pine Ridge Association

BEST TIMES March through May

AGENCY Henry W. Coe State Park, (408) 779-2728, **www.coepark.org**

PERMIT A first-come, first-served backcountry permit, available at the park visitor center, is required. Space is almost always available.

Highlights
Located in the heart of the Diablo Range, vast Henry W. Coe State Park features soaring ridges, steep canyons, gurgling creeks, thriving oaks, abundant wildlife, radiant spring wildflowers, and the immortal words etched on the monument to Henry W. Coe—MAY THESE QUIET HILLS BRING PEACE TO THE SOULS OF THOSE WHO ARE SEEKING. Encompassing more than 87,000 acres, it is the largest state park in Northern California—and provides unparalleled backcountry opportunities.

Hike Overview
The convoluted drainage of Coyote Creek surrounds the main park entrance area atop Pine Ridge. A mosaic of streams flowing through shady canyons, the watershed can be accessed via several steep trails from the main park entrance area. This journey tours some of the best features of the Western Zone: Pine Ridge, three different trail camps, two forks of Coyote Creek, and the perennial swimming waters of China Hole.

Beginning at the main park entrance, the hike travels along Pine Ridge before plummeting more than 1,000 feet to reach China Hole Trail Camp by Coyote Creek. After winding through The Narrows, a thin gap carved by the East Fork, the hike reaches Los Cruzeros Trail Camp. Returning, the route winds over open hillsides, passes Middle Fork Coyote Creek and Poverty Flat Trail Camp, and then climbs steeply back up Pine Ridge. The journey may be reduced by more than 2 miles via a connector trail between Poverty Flat and China Hole on Creekside Trail, an option that skips both The Narrows and Los Cruzeros Trail Camp.

Unlike most trips in Henry Coe, this adventure can be tackled in any season because water is present year-round—though the scorching heat of summer and early fall can be oppressive. The *Henry W. Coe State Park Trail and Camping Map* is strongly recommended as a complement to the maps in this book. It covers the entire park and all its trails and is available at the park visitor center or can be ordered from the Pine Ridge Association, the park's nonprofit partner (**www.coepark.org**).

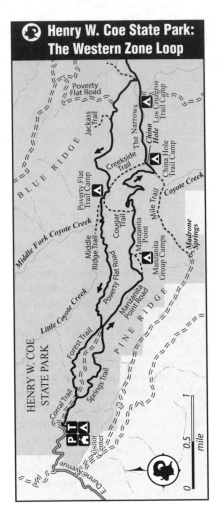

Henry W. Coe State Park: The Western Zone Loop

Trail Camps

A backcountry permit is required and must be obtained the day of your departure. All trail camp and backcountry permits are first-come, first-served—reservations are *not* accepted—and there is a fee of $5 per night per person. Quotas for each zone are seldom met; securing a backcountry permit is rarely an issue. Obtain your permit from the visitor center.

This hike visits three of the 19 designated trail camps in Henry Coe's Western Zone: China Hole, Los Cruzeros, and Poverty Flat. They are among the most popular in the park, and occasionally fill on busy weekends, especially on Memorial Day weekend. If space is unavailable, you can still camp in the Blue Ridge Zone—where camping is unrestricted—readily accessed a short distance upstream from Los Cruzeros Trail Camp.

Los Cruzeros Trail Camp, at the midpoint of the hike, neatly divides the trip into two equal segments. Three well-spaced sites are available near East Fork Coyote Creek, though none are great summer destinations; there is minimal shade and the adjacent section of creek usually dries up by June.

China Hole Trail Camp features one site near a small sandy beach on the banks of Coyote Creek. Located 100 feet downstream from its namesake swimming hole, the small camp has access to water year-round. The creek can turn somewhat green in late summer and fall—a filter is recommended. This is not the most secluded place to camp; China Hole is a popular destination, especially on weekends.

Poverty Flat Trail Camp features five sites along the banks of Middle Fork Coyote Creek. Several sites have picnic tables, and there is a centrally located outhouse. Poverty Flat is shaded during the hot summer months; water is often available from the creek through July and some upstream pools typically remain into fall.

Manzanita Group Camps are located 2 miles from the trailhead and available for group reservations ($75, **www. reserveamerica.com,** 1-800-444-7275). Ten sites are available.

Dogs and wood fires are prohibited. Campstoves permitted, except in times of extreme wildfire risk.

Getting There

Take Highway 101 to Morgan Hill and exit on East Dunne Avenue. Head east and follow East Dunne Avenue for 13 miles to the visitor center parking lot at road's end. After leaving the residential area of Morgan Hill, the road narrows to a twisting, exciting ascent. Located in a reconstructed ranch building at the main park entrance, the Henry Coe visitor center houses an excellent bookstore, sells state park maps and all the USGS quads for the area, and offers extensive literature about the park's natural history. The visitor center is open spring and summer weekends, 8 a.m.–4p.m., and sporadically on other days and during fall and winter.

Hiking It

The route begins across the road from the visitor center on single-track Corral Trail (0.0/2,650'). After crossing a small bridge, the trail contours into a lush world of black oak, bay trees, buckeyes, snowberry bushes, and coast live oaks. It then winds above precipitous slopes before encountering the first big-berry manzanita of the trip. Dozens of manzanita varieties exist, but few approach the massive size of these specimens; their twisting, blood-red trunks are almost treelike in girth. Chamise, toyon, and honeysuckle vines—common members of the park's chaparral community—appear alongside.

The trail breaks out into open hillsides graced with large valley oaks and soon reaches a six-way junction at Manzanita Point Road (0.6/2,510'). Cross the wide road, grab an interpretive brochure from the post, and continue on Forest Trail. (Adjacent Springs Trail and Manzanita Point Road both reconnect in a mile and are alternate routes for the return journey.) Forest Trail has numbered markers (corresponding to descriptions in the free brochure) that highlight many of the park's common trees and shrubs. After contouring through this shady educational world, rejoin Manzanita Point Road (1.8/2,330') at its junction with Springs Trail and Poverty Flat Road.

Bear left on wide Manzanita Point Road as it undulates along the ridgetop past valley oaks and ponderosa pines. The road then passes the pleasant Manzanita Group Camps before reaching China Hole and Madrone Spring trails just past Sites 6 and 7 (2.6/2,260').

BACKPACKING IN HENRY COE: ARE YOU PREPARED?

The park's endless succession of deep valleys hemmed by steep ridges makes for extremely strenuous hiking. Most backpacking trips require several thousand feet of elevation change on often challenging trails, and good fitness is required for any overnight trip. From late May through the first rains of winter, water is scarce in the park; a few perennial sources remain in the western regions, but most backcountry sources disappear by June. Longer backpacking trips are generally not recommended in summer or fall because of baking temperatures (often in the 90s), miles of unshaded trail, and little to no water.

Turn left on China Hole Trail to begin the descent.

China Hole Trail initially contours below the last group sites (a spur trail splits right to Site 9), passing some final ponderosa pines that give way to black oak, madrone, and blue oak. Soon the trail dives steeply through a corridor of massive big-berry manzanita (this unusual forest of skeletal fingers gives Manzanita Point its name) and later a zone burned by prescribed fire (a posted sign tells the story). Here manzanita diminishes, and thick chamise and buckbrush thrive on the regenerating hillside. The low-lying vegetation offers good views below of the Coyote Creek watershed and its multiple

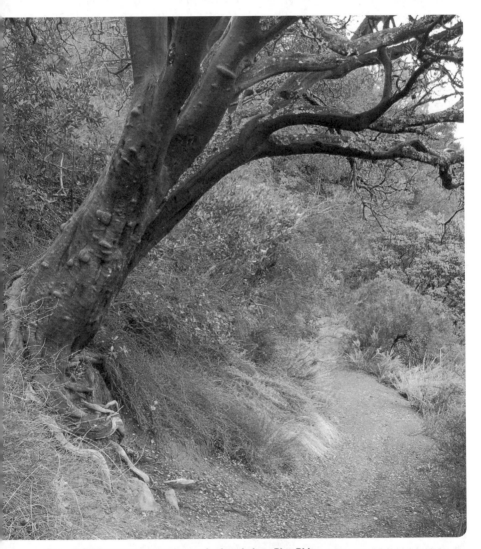

Tree-sized big-berry manzanita can be found along Pine Ridge.

drainages. California sage and sticky monkeyflower appear in the chaparral mix as the trail next encounters Manzanita Point and the junction with Cougar Trail (3.7/1,910').

Continue straight on China Hole Trail to begin a series of long, descending switchbacks to the canyon bottom and the junction with Mile Trail (5.2/1,150'). (As you head downward, note the marked ecological difference between the sun-exposed southern slopes of chaparral and shadier north slopes of oak woodland.) To reach China Hole Trail Camp, bear left (upstream) to cross the creek and quickly switchback roughly 30 feet above the water. Bear left on the obvious use trail and descend to the pleasant site.

To continue the journey from the junction with Mile Trail, proceed a short distance upstream. In summer and fall this stream is the only reliable water source on the hike, so fill your bottles. It's also a pleasant swimming hole. After a refreshing dip, continue upstream to quickly reach the confluence of Coyote Creek's Middle Fork (left) and East Fork (right). China Hole and Poverty Flat trail camps are connected via Creekside Trail along the Middle Fork, a shorter return option. To reach Los Cruzeros Trail Camp and complete the full Western Zone loop, bear right up the East Fork and enter the lush world of The Narrows.

There is no officially maintained trail through The Narrows, but a path is generally obvious and closely parallels the creek. This route requires crossing the stream in several places, and, depending on season and flow, may be a rock-hop or knee-deep ford. In times of heavy rains The Narrows may become impassable—*use caution*.

Profuse spring wildflowers color the ground beneath bay trees, willows, alders, and sycamores in this canyon environment, and soon you reach wide Mahoney Meadows Road and the first site of Los Cruzeros Trail Camp near the confluence of East Fork Coyote and Kelly creeks (6.2/1,230'). Bear left on Mahoney Meadows Road to bypass the second site (upstream and out of sight from the road on a curve of East Fork Coyote Creek) and reach the third site at the northern Mahoney Meadows Road creek crossing. If these are full, unrestricted camping is available a quarter mile upstream from Mahoney Meadows Road, beyond the boundary of Blue Ridge Zone.

The junction with Willow Ridge Trail (6.3/1,230') is located upstream on the right, just past the third site. To head back toward Pine Ridge, follow wide Mahoney Meadows Road north as it rock-hops the creek and climbs steeply through open woodland of blue oak and gray pine. Turn left at the junction with broad Poverty Flat Road (6.8/1,620') and remain on Poverty Flat Road as it ascends to reach Jackass Trail (7.0/1,790') before gently descending to a saddle below Jackass Peak (1,784'). From here, a short side trip leads to the level summit and its near-360-degree views. Several forks of Coyote Creek are visible below.

Poverty Flat Road plummets past this point to reach Middle Fork Coyote Creek and Creekside Trail (8.2/1,150'), which arrives from China Hole. The vegetation is lush once again; black oak and bay trees thrive, and the wide streambed of sycamores is a pleasant backdrop to Poverty Flat Trail Camp. Poverty Flat's five sites are spread along the stream close to the road: Site 5 by the Creekside Trail junction; Sites 3 and 4 by the outhouse and junction with Cougar Trail (8.3/1,160'); Site 2 by the creek crossing; and Site 1 just upstream from the Middle Ridge Trail junction (8.5/1,240').

To continue, remain on Poverty Flat Road as it begins a steady thousand-foot ascent along the flanks of Pine Ridge. (It is also possible to return via Manzanita Point and China Hole Trail by following Cougar Trail south from Poverty Flat. This single-track variation adds a mile to the journey.) Poverty Flat Road contours gently and sometimes ascends steeply for short, strenuous sections through a lush environment marked by the presence of black oak, buckeye, madrones, and spring wildflowers. An intense switchbacking climb at the end finally deposits you back on top of Pine Ridge at the earlier junction with Manzanita Point Road (10.2/2,330').

From here you can return on a different route by following Springs Trail as it travels along the margin of open oak woodland and past several dribbling springs to reach Corral Trail (11.5/2,510') and the final section back to the visitor center (12.1/2,650').

Giving Back

The **Pine Ridge Association** assists park staff in designing interpretive materials and presenting educational programs to the public. It offers a volunteer training program. Contact the association or learn more at (408) 779-2728 or **www.coepark.org**.

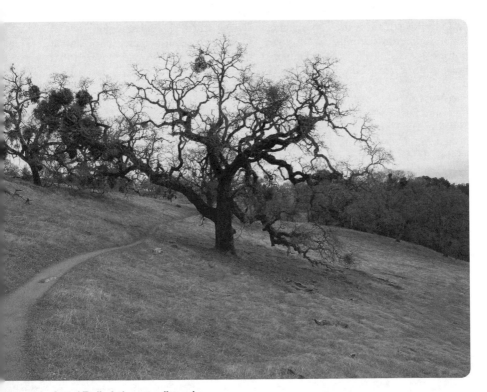

Corral Trail winds past valley oaks.

25 Henry W. Coe State Park:
MISSISSIPPI LAKE AND BEYOND

RATINGS	Scenery **7** Difficulty **10** Solitude **10**
ROUND-TRIP DISTANCE	24 miles (3–4 days) to Mississippi Lake 50+ miles (5–7 days) to Orestimba Wilderness
ELEVATION GAIN/LOSS	+6,000'/–6,000' to Mississippi Lake +9,500'/–9,500' to Orestimba Wilderness
RECOMMENDED MAP	*Henry W. Coe State Park Trail and Camping Map* by the Pine Ridge Association
BEST TIMES	March through May
AGENCY	Henry W. Coe State Park, (408) 779-2728, **www.coepark.org**
PERMIT	A first-come, first-served backcountry permit, available at the park visitor center, is required. Space is almost always available.

Highlights

Journey to the most remote wilderness in the Bay Area. To reach vast and distant Orestimba Wilderness, you must first hike more than 15 miles across some of the Bay Area's most rugged terrain. It's another 15 arduous miles back out. In between, stay as long as you possibly can in this seldom-visited wilderness area. It's an epic.

En route, in the middle of the park, is Mississippi Lake. At nearly a mile long, it's the park's largest lake and home to a sizeable population of largemouth bass. The surrounding blue oak woodland and a pleasant lakeshore site make this haven a worthwhile trip in its own right.

Hike Overview

Beginning at the main park entrance, the hike travels along Pine Ridge before plummeting more than 1,000 feet to reach China Hole Trail Camp by Coyote Creek. After winding through The Narrows, a thin gap carved by the East Fork, the hike reaches Los Cru-

zeros Trail Camp. The journey then climbs Willow Ridge to travel its long roller-coaster ridgeline to Mississippi Lake. Beyond the lake, the route drops into the Orestimba Creek watershed and embarks on a 20-mile loop around Robison Mountain in Orestimba Wilderness. The most straightforward return option is to retrace your steps, but other routes are available—ask park staff about using County Line and Bear Mountain roads.

A journey into Orestimba Wilderness requires excellent fitness, considerable self-reliance, and good map-reading and route-finding skills. Trails are often overgrown, unsigned, and/or indistinct; bushwhacking is occasionally necessary. Know what you're doing and be prepared for the unexpected.

Creeks in Orestimba Wilderness flow throughout winter and spring, but usually dry up by the end of May. Check with park staff about water availability if you are planning a late-spring excursion.

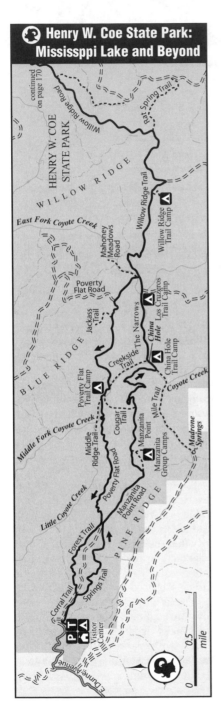

Henry W. Coe State Park: Mississppi Lake and Beyond

continued on page 170

Trail Camps

A backcountry permit is required and must be obtained the day of your departure. All trail camp and backcountry permits are first-come, first-served—reservations are *not* accepted—and there is a fee of $5 per night per person. Quotas for each zone are seldom met; securing a backcountry permit is rarely an issue. Obtain your permit from the visitor center.

This backpacking trip visits the Western, Interior, Mississippi, and Orestimba Wilderness backcountry zones. Camping is permitted anywhere outside of the Western Zone and its designated trail campsites. Recommended overnight spots in the Western Zone (your approach route) are **Los Cruzeros** and **Willow Ridge** (described below). In the event these trail camps are full, **Blue Ridge Zone** (and its unrestricted camping) can be readily accessed a short distance upstream from Los Cruzeros. It is possible to reach Mississippi Lake in one day, though it is an arduous 12-mile hike. Good campsites are abundant throughout **Orestimba Wilderness.**

Getting There

Take Highway 101 to Morgan Hill and exit on East Dunne Avenue. Head east and follow East Dunne Avenue for 13 miles to the visitor center parking lot at road's end. After leaving the residential area of Morgan Hill, the road narrows to a twisting, exciting ascent. Located in a reconstructed ranch building at the main park entrance, the Henry Coe visitor center houses an excellent bookstore, sells state park maps and all the USGS quads for the area, and offers extensive literature about the park's natural history. The visitor center is open spring and summer weekends,

🧭 Henry W. Coe State Park: Mississippi Lake and Beyond

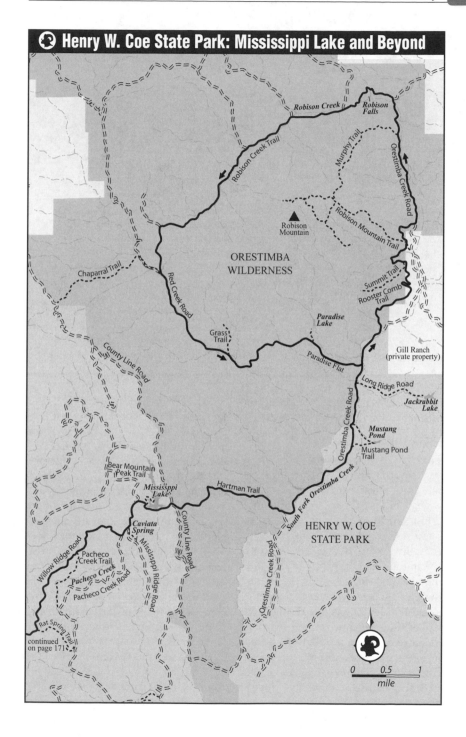

Robison Creek

Robison Falls

Robison Creek Trail

Murphy Trail

Orestimba Creek Road

Robison Mountain

Robison Mountain Trail

ORESTIMBA WILDERNESS

Chaparral Trail

Red Creek Road

Summit Trail

Rooster Comb Trail

Paradise Lake

Grass Trail

Paradise Flat

Gill Ranch (private property)

County Line Road

Long Ridge Road

Jackrabbit Lake

Mustang Pond

Mustang Pond Trail

Orestimba Creek Road

Bear Mountain Peak Trail

Mississippi Lake

Hartman Trail

South Fork Orestimba Creek

HENRY W. COE STATE PARK

Caviata Spring

County Line Road

Willow Ridge Road

Pacheco Creek Trail

Mississippi Ridge Road

Pacheco Creek

Pacheco Creek Road

Orestimba Creek Road

Rat Spring Trail

continued on page 171

0   0.5   1
mile

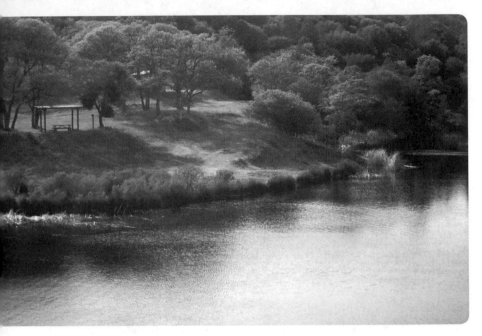

Mississippi Lake campsite

from 8 a.m.–4 p.m., and sporadically on other days and during fall and winter.

Hiking It

The route begins across the road from the visitor center on single-track Corral Trail (0.0/2,650'). After crossing a small bridge, the trail contours into a lush world of black oak, bay trees, buckeyes, snowberry bushes, and coast live oaks. It then winds above precipitous slopes before encountering the first big-berry manzanita of the trip. Dozens of manzanita varieties exist, but few approach the massive size of these specimens; their twisting, blood-red trunks are almost treelike in girth. Chamise, toyon, and honeysuckle vines—common members of the park's chaparral community—appear alongside.

The trail breaks out into open hillsides graced with large valley oaks and soon reaches a six-way junction at Manzanita Point Road (0.6/2,510'). Cross the wide road, grab an interpretive brochure from the post, and continue on Forest Trail. (Adjacent Springs Trail and Manzanita Point Road both reconnect in a mile and are alternate routes for the return journey.) Forest Trail has numbered markers (corresponding to descriptions in the free brochure) that highlight many of the park's common trees and shrubs. After contouring through this shady educational world, rejoin Manzanita Point Road (1.8/2,330') at its junction with Springs Trail and Poverty Flat Road.

Bear left on wide Manzanita Point Road as it undulates along the ridgetop past valley oaks and ponderosa pines.

The road then passes the pleasant Manzanita Group Camps before reaching China Hole and Madrone Spring trails just past Sites 6 and 7 (2.6/2,260'). Turn left on China Hole Trail to begin the descent.

China Hole Trail initially contours below the last group sites (a spur trail splits right to Site 9), passing some final ponderosa pines that give way to black oak, madrone, and blue oak. Soon the trail dives steeply through a corridor of massive big-berry manzanita (this unusual forest of skeletal fingers gives Manzanita Point its name) and later a zone burned by prescribed fire (a posted sign tells the story). Here manzanita diminishes, and thick chamise and buckbrush thrive on the regenerating hillside. The low-lying vegetation offers good views below of the Coyote Creek watershed and its multiple drainages. California sage and sticky monkeyflower appear in the chaparral mix as the trail next encounters Manzanita Point and the junction with Cougar Trail (3.7/1,910').

Continue straight on China Hole Trail to begin a series of long, descending switchbacks to the canyon bottom and the junction with Mile Trail (5.2/1,150'). (As you head downward, note the marked ecological difference between the sun-exposed southern slopes of chaparral and shadier north slopes of oak woodland.) To reach China Hole Trail Camp, bear left (upstream) to cross the creek and quickly switchback roughly 30 feet above the water. Bear left on the obvious use trail and descend to the pleasant site.

To continue the journey from the junction with Mile Trail, proceed a short distance upstream. In summer and fall this stream is the only reliable water source on the hike, so fill your bottles. It's also a pleasant swimming hole. After a refreshing dip, continue upstream to quickly reach the confluence of Coyote Creek's Middle Fork (left) and East Fork (right). Bear right up the East Fork and enter the lush world of The Narrows.

There is no officially maintained trail through The Narrows, but a path is generally obvious and closely parallels the creek. This route requires crossing the stream in several places, and, depending on season and flow, may be a rock-hop or knee-deep ford. In times of heavy rains The Narrows may become impassable—*use caution.*

Profuse spring wildflowers color the ground beneath bay trees, willows, alders, and sycamores in this canyon environment, and soon you reach wide Mahoney Meadows Road and the first site of Los Cruzeros Trail Camp near the confluence of East Fork Coyote and Kelly creeks (6.2/1,230'). Bear left on Mahoney Meadows Road to bypass the second site (upstream and out of sight from the road on a curve of East Fork Coyote Creek) and reach the third site at the northern Mahoney Meadows Road creek crossing. If these are full, unrestricted camping is available a quarter mile upstream from Mahoney Meadows Road, beyond the boundary of Blue Ridge Zone.

Before leaving camp, fill your water bottles at adjacent Coyote Creek, the last reliable source for the next 6 miles. Strike out on single-track Willow Ridge Trail (6.3/1,230'), located to the right just past the northern Mahoney Meadows Road creek crossing. Willow Ridge Trail momentarily drops to the creekbed, then begins a climbing traverse up the ridge. Black oaks appear as you wind along the oak woodland and chaparral margin and then descend briefly on a shadier north slope marked by bay trees and coffee berry.

Climbing again, the route obtains the ridgeline and begins a more direct ascent. Broken-down barbed wire fence appears in places, relics of the land's ranching days.

The trail climbs relentlessly along the ridgeline, alternating between black-oak shade and scratchy chaparral. Near the top is a junction on the right for Willow Ridge Trail Camp (7.5/2,190'), located 0.2 mile down this thin trail past Willow Ridge Spring. Blue oak, gray pine, and coast live oak provide shade for several grassy clearings with excellent views of ridges to the west. Nearby Willow Ridge Spring is, however, unreliable—bring sufficient water if staying the night.

Continuing, you soon attain the top of Willow Ridge (7.8/2,400'); turn left onto Willow Ridge Road. For the next 4 miles, the route follows the dry and exposed ridgeline as it endlessly undulates through chamise-dominated chaparral. You are now entering the western edge of the 2007 Lick Fire, which burned half the park, including almost all of Orestimba Wilderness. Extensive brush was cleared along the south side of the road as a potential fire break. You'll see evidence of the conflagration for the remainder of your journey, though the landscape is regenerating rapidly.

Willow Ridge also marks the divide between the Coyote Creek and Pacheco Creek watersheds, and provides far-reaching views. From the junction with Eagle Pines Trail (8.2/2,610'), vast stretches of the park spread out below. East Fork Coyote Creek flows through a linear valley to the north, the massif of Bear Mountain and its ridges is visible northeast (the most severely burned portion of the park during the Lick Fire), and Willow Ridge Road can be seen snaking northeast toward hidden Mississippi Lake. Continue hiking on Willow Ridge Road as it drops steeply to reach Rat Spring Trail on the right (8.6/2,450'). (Unreliable Rat Spring is located on a spur trail 0.3 mile down Rat Spring Trail; a better option is Caviata Spring 3 miles ahead.)

Wild cucumber vines, yerba santa, abundant poison oak, coyote brush, buckbrush, and manzanita add variety to the chaparral as you continue along the ridgeline. The roller coaster grinds onward as you pass several trails joining from the right—Pacheco Creek Trail (10.3/2,250'), Pacheco Ridge Road (11.2/2,470'), and Mississippi Ridge Road (11.4/2,400'). To reach nearby Caviata Spring, bear right on Mississippi Ridge Road and then quickly left on a 0.2-mile spur trail.

From here the route finally descends to the lake, passing Bear Mountain Peak Trail on the left (11.8/2,250') before reaching the junction with Mississippi Lake Dam Road (12.0/2,150'). To reach the nearby established picnic site (tables and shade), bear left to remain on Willow Ridge Road; the site is 0.2 mile ahead by the lakeshore. To continue toward Orestimba Wilderness, turn right and descend to the southern lakeshore on the dam road.

Surrounded by thriving oak woodland, Mississippi Lake is an oasis in an otherwise dry landscape. Turtles, rabbits, birds, and other wildlife are abundant. The 0.7-mile-long lake can be circumnavigated (a 3-mile loop) in search of campsites and fishing spots. Good sites are scattered throughout, but thick shrubbery and poison oak make lakeshore access difficult. Outhouses are located near the dam and at the lake's northern end. Bass fishing is excellent.

You may want to fill up water bottles before continuing; the lake is your

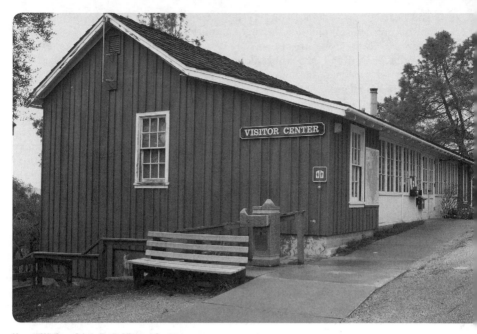

Henry W. Coe State Park Visitor Center

only source for the next 2.5 miles. To head toward Orestimba Wilderness, follow well-graded Mississippi Dam Road past the lake's southern shore to reach County Line Road (12.5/2,180'). Turn right to quickly find Hartman Trail on the left (12.6/2,210'). County Line Road marks the watershed divide between Pacheco Creek, which ultimately flows west into the Bay, and Orestimba Creek, which heads east into the Central Valley. The road also travels the border between Santa Clara and Stanislaus counties and defines the western boundary of Orestimba Wilderness.

Hartman Trail is thin and sometimes indistinct. From County Line Road, it immediately drops through oaks and chaparral to reach a small saddle before climbing to the top of a promontory (2,210') with good views northeast. Robison Mountain (2,656') and Orestimba Wilderness are clearly visible; the rocky outcrop of Rooster Comb can be spotted on Robison's eastern flanks. The trail curves briefly north, then turns right and drops steeply through a dense chamise corridor. The route reenters full oak woodland as the trail reaches a barbed wire fence above a small gully at 1,400 feet. The path becomes increasingly indistinct— if you lose the trail, follow the drainage downward to reach Orestimba Creek Road (14.7/1,170').

Campsites are abundant in the broad, delightful valley of Orestimba Creek. One good overnight option is Kingbird Pond, tucked away 1.2 miles south of Hartman Trail; follow Orestimba Creek Road south for 0.7 mile and bear left on Kingbird Pond Trail. If you are not stopping for the night, continue north (downstream) on Orestimba Creek Road as it winds along the broad creekbed through vibrant blue oak woodland.

The level hiking here is pleasant compared to the strenuous route in. Also, you can eschew the wide road and travel directly along the banks of Orestimba Creek, a pleasant cross-country route. A mile north of Hartman Trail, the road deviates slightly from the creek. Opt for the off-trail streamside route, unless you're interested in exploring Mustang Pond. Accessed via half-mile Mustang Pond Trail, the small lake can be reached from Orestimba Creek Road at a southern junction (16.2/1,210') and a northern junction (16.6/1,170').

Red Creek joins Orestimba Creek immediately upstream from the northern junction for Mustang Pond. After crossing the creek, the winding road leaves and then returns to the waterway before reaching Long Ridge Road on the right (17.3/1,100'). (Long Ridge Road leads to another pond, Jackrabbit Lake, 1.6 miles to the east. If you want to enjoy this side trip, be sure to bear left at the fork 1.2 miles out. The lake covers 6 acres in spring but diminishes in summer and fall.)

A short 0.3 mile beyond Long Ridge Road you pass Red Creek Road on the left (17.6/1,070')—your return route. (Paradise Flat—an idyllic picnic or camping spot—is a short distance west along lower Red Creek Road.) The loop around Robison Mountain begins at this point, as Orestimba Creek Road continues downstream to reach Rooster Comb Trail on the left (18.2/1,060'). Orestimba Creek Road continues through the private property of Gill Ranch; follow single-track Rooster Comb Trail to stay inside the park.

Rooster Comb Trail becomes overgrown and indistinct in places, but begins climbing through open blue oak woodland to steadily traverse the slopes above Gill Ranch. As you round the eastern corner of Rooster Comb, the trail becomes rockier. Chaparral now predominates—chamise, sticky monkeyflower, scrub oak, and poison oak are common. You pass the posted trail to Rooster Comb Summit on the left (20.0/1,250') and descend into Lion Canyon, switchbacking near the bottom to cross an ephemeral trickle. Leaving the narrow canyon, the trail continues north and traverses the slopes above the park boundary. It then passes faint Robison Mountain Trail on the left (20.8/1,150') and winds above the property fence and a small reservoir before descending to rejoin Orestimba Creek Road (21.3/1,050').

The level valley of Orestimba Creek now reaches nearly a quarter mile in width. Orestimba Creek Road travels along the valley's western margin and offers easy walking. The off-trail route along the stream is more dramatic, however. Enormous California sycamores line the rocky streambed, their roots feeding into the water like giant hoses. Blue oak woodland lines either side of the valley as do a few outlying valley oaks. The Robison Creek drainage is apparent ahead, tracing from the west. Bear left on Robison Creek Trail beyond the confluence of Orestimba and Robison creeks (23.2/940') and head west below Robison Mountain's northern flanks. Anglers may continue 0.7 mile downstream from the confluence along Orestimba Creek to reach the park's northeastern boundary. Trout are reportedly present along this section of creek, though you may have to fish for a long, long time to find one.

Robison Trail is a wide, grassy road that initially climbs above hidden Robison Creek. The trail cuts deeply into the hillside to traverse around a small tributary; secretive Robison Falls is located immediately upstream from this tributary's confluence with Robison Creek. (It is possible to come within earshot by descending off-trail past the tributary, but large rock outcrops and steep slopes preclude reaching Robison Creek itself. The falls are best reached by dropping down before you reach the tributary or by traveling directly along Robison Creek above its confluence with Orestimba Creek.)

Robison Trail eventually drops to reach Robison Creek in a narrow riparian canyon, flush with buckeyes, poison oak, and gray pines. After crossing the small creek, the trail fades into grass, recrosses the creek several more times, and then suddenly enters an open field studded with huge sycamores and good campsites. Shortly past this meadow, Pinto Creek and Trail join Robison Creek from the north in a Sierra-esque conifer landscape of large gray pines (25.2/1,180'). A scrambling side-trip up overgrown Pinto Creek rewards with a secluded swimming hole.

Beyond Pinto Creek, Robison Creek Trail becomes more apparent as the canyon gradually narrows. The trail crosses a significant tributary (as large

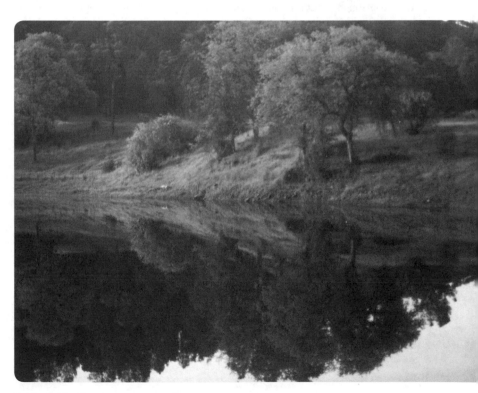

Outdoor reflection

as the main creek) and then becomes only intermittently visible—stay close to the creek. As the ever-narrowing canyon bends west, the trail turns up a wash gully on the south slopes. Traversing upward, the obvious road soon attains the ridgeline divide between Robison and Red creeks (27.6/1,580'). Good views appear once again as the Red Creek valley opens up below.

After savoring the view, bear right along the ridgeline on an overgrown and unnamed, but easy-to-follow road to the top of the nearby knoll (1,767'). Two roads join here—bear left to begin the steep ridgeline descent into the valley. The trail passes a small pond shortly before reaching Red Creek Road (28.8/1,270').

Red Creek Road marks the final leg of the Robison Mountain loop. The long spine of Bear Mountain (2,604') rises southwest above the valley and defines the high ridge margin of the Red Creek watershed. Your route heads downstream (south) along Red Creek, where the wide trail passes through a narrow valley lined with blue oaks and seasonally covered with the round, tufted flowers of purple owl's clover. The valley widens noticeably as you pass Grass Trail on the left (30.5/1,210') and then curve north to wind over low-lying foothills. After a steady but gradual ascent, the road descends to a small tributary and enters Paradise Flat.

Site of an old landing strip, aptly named Paradise Flat is a massive field of blue oak savanna more than a mile long. Grass and spring wildflowers flourish in this idyllic landscape, which makes an ideal final stop on the circuit around Robison Mountain. Shady campsites are everywhere, and seasonal water is often available from the two

THE 2007 LICK FIRE

In early September 2007, a human-caused conflagration (begun by an illegal and poorly maintained burn barrel on private property) consumed 47,760 acres, most of it within Henry Coe State Park. Known as the Lick Fire, it burned most of the northern half of the park, including all of Orestimba Wilderness. It extended south to the edge of Kelly and Coit lakes and west to Mississippi Ridge above Los Cruzeros Trail Camp. Its intensity varied dramatically, however, leaving much of the park's trees and woodlands mostly unscathed. Areas of chaparral, most notably thick chamise, burned more severely. The slopes of Bear Mountain were particularly charred. Trails were largely unaffected.

Fire is a natural and recurring process in the region, and the landscape is quickly recovering. Other than some blackened trunks, you may not even notice its effects in many areas. In other places, the skeletal fingers of fire-seared manzanita and chamise poke out from the regenerating chaparral. The fire also provides a unique opportunity to study the effects of wildfire on the landscape. Learn more at **www.coefire2007. info**, where you can view maps of the fire, pictures of its immediate aftermath, and panoramic images of recovering areas.

small creeks that border the area to the north and south. Red Creek Road travels along the flat's northern edge, reaching the junction for Paradise Lake shortly after curving back eastward (32.2/1,250').

Paradise Lake is only 0.3 mile from Red Creek Road and abuts the rocky southern flanks of Robison Mountain. The snags protruding from the lake belie its artificial nature but the setting is pleasant and the scenery excellent. Back on Red Creek Road, you soon return to Orestimba Creek Road to complete the loop around Robison Mountain (33.1/1,170'). From here, the long journey home begins. The most direct route retraces your route for 11.4 miles past Mississippi Lake to Los Cruzeros Trail Camp via Orestimba Creek Road, Hartman Trail, and Willow Ridge Road and Trail. (The state park map reveals several alternative routes back to Los Cruzeros, but they all require more effort.)

From Los Cruzeros (44.6/1,230), you can continue to retrace your earlier route back to Pine Ridge, though the following return route is 0.7 mile shorter and adds variety to the end of your trip. To take this route, follow wide Mahoney Meadows Road north as it rock-hops the creek and climbs steeply through open woodland of blue oak and gray pine. Turn left at the junction with broad Poverty Flat Road (45.0/1,620') and remain on Poverty Flat Road as it ascends to reach Jackass Trail (45.2/1,790') before gently descending to a saddle below Jackass Peak (1,784'). From here, a short side trip leads to the level summit and its near-360-degree views. Several forks of Coyote Creek are visible below.

Poverty Flat Road plummets past this point to reach Middle Fork Coyote Creek and Creekside Trail (46.4/1,150'),

which arrives from China Hole. The vegetation is lush once again; black oak and bay trees thrive, and the wide streambed of sycamores is a pleasant backdrop to Poverty Flat Trail Camp. Poverty Flat's five sites are spread along the stream close to the road: site 5 by the Creekside Trail junction; Sites 3 and 4 by the outhouse and junction with Cougar Trail (46.5/1,160'); Site 2 by the creek crossing; and Site 1 just upstream from the Middle Ridge Trail junction (46.7/1,240').

To continue, remain on Poverty Flat Road as it begins a steady thousand-foot ascent along the flanks of Pine Ridge. (It is also possible to return via Manzanita Point and China Hole Trail by following Cougar Trail south from Poverty Flat. This single-track variation adds a mile to the journey.) Poverty Flat Road contours gently and sometimes ascends steeply for short, strenuous sections through a lush environment marked by the presence of black oak, buckeye, madrones, and spring wildflowers. An intense switchbacking climb at the end finally deposits you back on top of Pine Ridge at the earlier junction with Manzanita Point Road (48.4/2,330').

From here you can return on a different route by following Springs Trail as it travels along the margin of open oak woodland and past several dribbling springs to reach Corral Trail (49.7/2,510') and the final section back to the visitor center (50.3/2,650').

Giving Back

The **Pine Ridge Association** assists park staff in designing interpretive materials and presenting educational programs to the public. It offers a volunteer training program. Contact the association or learn more at (408) 779-2728 or **www.coepark.org**.

26 Henry W. Coe State Park:
COIT LAKE AND VICINITY

RATINGS	Scenery **7** Difficulty **7** Solitude **8**
ROUND-TRIP DISTANCE	12.4 miles
ELEVATION GAIN/LOSS	+3,800'/–3,800'
RECOMMENDED MAP	Henry W. Coe State Park Trail and Camping Map by the Pine Ridge Association
BEST TIMES	March through May
AGENCY	Henry W. Coe State Park, (408) 779-2728, **www.coepark.org**
PERMIT	A first-come, first-served backcountry permit, available at the park visitor center, is required. Space is almost always available.

Highlights
The rising bulwark of Wasno Ridge, a heart-pumping obstacle that keeps hiking traffic to a minimum, guards the approach to Henry Coe's southern backcountry. Kelly and Coit lakes await beyond, ideal base camps for further exploration. Several small ponds, seldom-trod creek valleys, a maze of trails, and hidden Pacheco Falls await discovery.

Hike Overview
The adventure begins from Coyote Creek Trailhead on Coe's southwestern edge, directly ascending Wasno Ridge on single-track Anza and Jackson trails. It then follows old ranch roads to Kelly Lake and then over Willow Ridge to Coit Lake. The return journey follows Dexter and Grizzly Gulch trails for a more gradual descent down Wasno Ridge. This journey makes for an excellent overnight trip, though the effort and scenery merit at least one extra day for exploration.

Water is readily available in season from Coyote Creek at the trailhead, and from several springs and ponds en route (a filter is recommended).

The hike can be completed year-round (Kelly and Coit lakes serve as reliable water sources), but baking heat, shadeless slopes, and increasingly funky water make this a less attractive option in summer and fall.

The Henry W. Coe State Park Trail and Camping Map is strongly recommended as a complement to the maps in this book. It covers the entire park and all its trails and is available at the park visitor center or can be ordered from the Pine Ridge Association, the park's nonprofit partner (**www.coepark.org**).

Trail Camps
A backcountry permit is required and must be obtained the day of your departure. All permits are first-come, first-served—reservations are *not* accepted—and there is a fee of $5 per night per person. Quotas for each zone are seldom met, and securing a backcountry permit is rarely an issue. Obtain your permit from the self-service station at nearby Hunting Hollow Trailhead (directions below).

This hike travels through (in order) the **Mahoney, Kelly, Coit,** and **Grizzly**

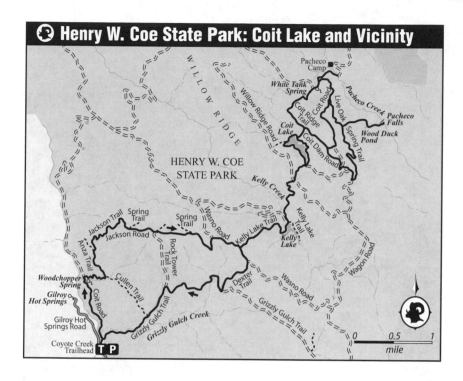

Henry W. Coe State Park: Coit Lake and Vicinity

Gulch backcountry zones. Camping is unrestricted in this region of the park. A few established sites and outhouses can be found around Coit and Kelly lakes; otherwise all camping is primitive. *Camping is prohibited within a half mile of the trailhead.* Woodchopper Spring is a mile from the trailhead and provides the closest, best option.

Getting There

Take the Leavesley Road exit from Highway 101 in Gilroy and follow Leavesley Road 1.8 miles east to New Avenue. Turn left and follow New Avenue 0.6 mile to Roop Road, and turn right. Roop Road becomes Gilroy Hot Springs Road and reaches Coyote Creek County Park on the left in 3.0 miles. Continue 3.0 miles past the park entrance to reach Hunting Hollow Trailhead on the right; stop here to ob-

tain your backcountry permit. Coyote Creek Trailhead is 1.7 miles farther at a bridge marking the farthest public access permitted on Gilroy Hot Springs Road. It is possible to park overnight here, though vandalism and theft have been reported. The park recommends leaving your vehicle at Hunting Hollow Trailhead.

Hiking It

From Coyote Creek Trailhead (0.0/940'), begin down wide Coit Road as it initially parallels the creek. You quickly meet Grizzly Gulch Trail (your return route), which joins from the right (0.1/960'). Continue on Coit Road to begin a slow climb that soon passes a fenced cattle-loading enclosure from past ranching days. The trail rises and descends, encountering large, big-berry manzanita and healthy

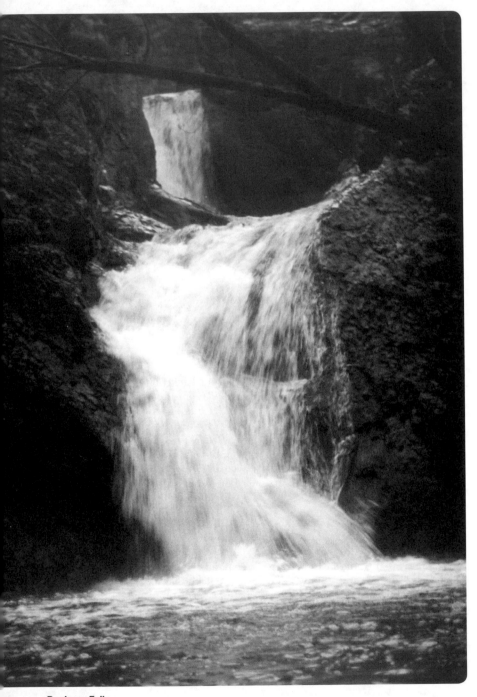

Pacheco Falls

valley oak. A giant rusting water tank indicates your approach to Anza Trail and Woodchopper Spring on the right (1.0/1,090').

The spring and its water faucet are located by the trail junction and provide a dependable source for much of the year (check with park staff in late summer and fall). Several shady campsites are also nearby. Also at the junction, an interpretive sign highlights the 1775–1776 Spanish expedition, led by Juan Bautista de Anza, that attempted (and failed) to find a route through this convoluted region. The Spaniards dubbed this area "Sierra del Chasco" ("Mountains of Deception"); they would be the last Europeans to visit the area for nearly a century.

Turning uphill on Anza Trail, you pass beneath bay trees and coast live oak as the shady single-track path switchbacks steadily upward to Cullen Trail on the right (1.6/1,440'). Bear left to remain on Anza Trail and traverse open slopes flush with spring wildflowers and good views. At the junction with Jackson Trail (1.9/1,560'), turn right to head toward Kelly Lake.

Views expand on the sustained ascent along Jackson Trail. Looking north, Pine Ridge and the main park entrance area are visible 6 miles away—tall and distinctive ponderosa pines can be identified on clear days. Beyond, Lick Observatory can be spotted atop Mt. Hamilton (4,213'). As the trail attains the Wasno ridgeline, views reach as far south as Fremont Peak (3,171') east of Monterey Bay, and beyond to the Santa Lucia Range of Big Sur. The trail next passes two small ponds and reaches the junction for seasonally dribbling Elderberry Spring (3.3/2,360').

Jackson Trail now widens to become Jackson Road as it hugs the ridgeline. The route passes a four-way junction for Rock Tower Trail (3.7/2,520') shortly before attaining the ridge's highest point (2,676'). Continue on Jackson Road, and begin a slow descent past hidden Spring Trail on the left (4.2/2,630'), then bank sharply left to reach Wasno Road (4.7/2,420'). Turn right to quickly encounter Kelly Lake Trail on the left (4.9/2,420').

Kelly Lake Trail first undulates through pleasant blue oak woodland studded with gray pines, but then plummets. Black and coast live oaks, bay and buckeye trees, and huge manzanita populate the shady slopes. Kelly Lake remains hidden from view until the very end, where the trail deposits you on the dam enclosing the northern shore.

Narrow Kelly Lake is enclosed by steep and brushy slopes, discouraging lakeshore camping and access. For better camping options, take the trail to the dam's north end and turn right on Kelly Lake Trail, which parallels the eastern lakeshore; a good camping area can be found above the lake's south end in the upper Kelly Creek drainage. Additional camping options are downstream near Kelly Creek below the dam; there are also a few small clearings tucked in the brush near the lakeshore. To continue on to Coit Lake, bear left at the northern end of the dam and then turn right on Coit Road by the outhouse (5.9/1,880').

Wide Coit Road initially climbs through a lush environment of varied oaks, bay trees, and buckeye before traversing more open slopes. Enjoy views of the Kelly Creek drainage below and Wasno Ridge above as the hillside becomes increasingly cloaked with chaparral. You crest southern Willow Ridge between Kelly and Coit lakes, which marks the divide between

The Natural History of Henry Coe: A Brief Survey

A series of long, high ridges defines the topography of Henry W. Coe State Park. Most trend in a north-south direction and trap moisture from east-moving storms. Each successive ridge to the east receives less precipitation, creating a marked precipitation gradient across the park. The park's western regions receive twice as much annual rain (25 to 30 inches) as those in the east (10 to 20 inches), a pattern that greatly affects the park's ecosystems.

The main park entrance area is located atop 2,500-foot Pine Ridge on the western edge of the park. This long ridge receives enough moisture to support a diverse oak woodland ecosystem (valley, black, and coast live oaks are common), which is joined by both gray pines and, oddly, tall ponderosa pines. Ponderosas are common throughout the Sierra Nevada foothills, but are found in only one other place in the Bay Area (Henry Cowell Redwoods State Park). On the eastern flanks of Pine Ridge, bay trees, madrone, buckeye, and a variety of ferns flourish on shady slopes. Pockets of chaparral appear on exposed hillsides, but are uncommon. Along the many forks of Coyote Creek below Pine Ridge grow California sycamores, drawing sustenance from the streambeds. Look for these water-loving trees at moist creeksides throughout the park. Poison oak is ubiquitous along Pine Ridge and throughout the park—be watchful!

Blue, Willow, and Rockhouse ridges rise progressively east of Pine Ridge, followed by the tall ridgeline of Bear Mountain (2,604'). They define the drier eastern margins of the Coyote Creek watershed and are cloaked with chaparral. Oak woodland species grow near valley bottoms, with hardy blue oaks and gray pines appearing in greatest

the Coyote Creek and Pacheco Creek watersheds. A four-way junction with Willow Ridge Road is met here (6.7/2,240')—continue straight on Coit Road. The trail then descends through young oaks rivaled in size by adjacent manzanita to reach the reedy southern shore of Coit Lake (7.0/2,080').

Coit Lake is ringed by easy trails. An established campsite and outhouse are located on the southwest shore; a few good sites (and another outhouse) are located by the dam on the lake's northern edge; and a grassy area resides near the fenced enclosure at Coit Lake Horse Camp on the eastern shore. A mix of blue oak, gray pine, coast live oak, manzanita, chamise, and coyote brush surround the lake, joined by abundant poison oak. While shore access is easier here than at Kelly Lake, there are only a few spots wide enough for fishing; try the area around the dam for your chance at the lake's numerous bass and crappie. Drinking water can usually be drawn from the outflow near the dam. Otherwise the lake is the only source.

abundance and surrounded by a wide variety of shrubs and wildflowers. In the chaparral, chamise and buckbrush predominate and provide little shade for hikers on long ridgetop traverses. This pattern repeats itself in the southern regions of the park, where Mahoney, Wasno, Willow, and Pacheco ridges define the topography.

Beyond Bear Mountain, in the northeast region of the park, the topography changes. Instead of a series of long ridges, singular Robison Mountain (2,656') dominates 23,300-acre Orestimba Wilderness. Three creeks—Red, Robison, and Orestimba—ring the massif. Flowing through broad valleys, they provide habitat for a wide but low-lying corridor of blue oak savanna. Large gray pines and creekside sycamores join this hardiest of oak species below the thick chaparral of higher elevations.

Temperature inversions are common in Henry Coe's deep valleys in winter and spring, with cooler air masses settling at lower elevations. This phenomenon is particularly evident in spring as higher valley slopes are already green with new leaves and flowers, while trees along the valley bottoms lag several weeks behind.

Birdlife is abundant in the park (137 species have been identified), and among the most audible are introduced wild turkeys that strut the woodlands searching for females in spring. You may frequently hear them gobbling in the trees. Male turkeys can be surprisingly aggressive—*use caution*. Large golden eagles, red-tailed hawks, and acorn woodpeckers are just a few of the other species that call the park home.

Mammals such as bobcats and mountain lions are common, preying on the park's numerous deer and small rodents. Nonnative wild pigs also are abundant. These large, black, hairy creatures search for food by rooting the ground with their snouts; their "pig tracks" are common throughout the park. They have poor eyesight and usually are quickly scared off.

There are many other campsites and delightful spots within a few miles of Coit Lake. Hoover Lake is 2.5 miles north along Willow Ridge Road. The drainage below Coit Lake Dam makes for fun off-trail exploration through open woodlands. But the recommended adventure is to Pacheco Creek and its seldom-visited waterfall, a 6-mile loop from Coit Lake with around 2,000 feet of elevation gain and loss. Additionally, those looking to spend the night deeper in the park should consider camping near small Wood Duck Pond, less than a half mile above the falls.

To reach the falls, proceed to Live Oak Spring Trail either via Coit Dam Road and then Coit Road from the north end of the lake, or via Coit Road from the south end of the lake. Live Oak Spring Trail splits and then rejoins as it traverses the slopes above Pacheco Creek canyon—take the lower option or risk missing the falls turnoff. Watch for the unmarked trail on the right to the falls, located just south of where Live Oak Spring Trail rejoins itself near two collapsed oak trees. The trail passes Wood Duck Pond as it descends a small ridgeline en route to the shady gorge below the falls. Roughly 200 feet above the creek, a spur trail splits left to reach vertical views into the rock chasm below.

The broad valley of Pacheco Creek above the falls also makes for idyllic camping and exploration. From Coit Lake's north end, follow Coit Dam Road and then Coit Ridge Trail past aptly named White Tank Spring to Coit Road and Pacheco Camp. From Coit Lake's south end, follow Coit Road all the way to Pacheco Camp. It's a 2- to 4-mile round-trip, depending on the route you choose.

After savoring Coit Lake and vicinity for as long as possible, you may be tempted to vary your return route to Kelly Lake Trail based on several alternate routes noted on the state park map. However, the most direct option is to retrace your steps on Coit Road to Kelly Lake Trail and its earlier junction with Wasno Road (9.1/2,420'). From there, the shortest route home descends into Grizzly Gulch to the south. Bear left on Wasno Road to quickly reach Dexter Trail on the right (9.3/2,420').

Descend on Dexter Trail through open blue oak woodlands, beyond a diminutive pond, and then drop steeply past increasing bay trees and coast live oak to reach the unsigned junction with Grizzly Gulch Trail (9.9/1,940'). Turn right on Grizzly Gulch Trail and traverse a moist creek gully and then contour shady slopes. At Rock Tower Trail (10.9/1,740'), you may take a short half-mile detour to the right and climb 250 feet uphill to reach another small pond ringed by impressive oaks.

Back on Grizzly Gulch Trail, the route begins a more direct descent above a narrow creek gully. Valley oak, buckeye, and madrone soon appear, indicative of the moist riparian environment. A few hundred feet from the bottom you pass the posted junction for indistinct Cullen Trail on the right (11.4/1,270'). Grizzly Gulch Trail descends into an increasingly lush world and soon reaches canyon bottom and crosses Grizzly Gulch Creek. Sycamores, ferns, and black oaks appear as the trail ascends and contours the slopes above the creek. It then passes Spike Jones Trail on the left (12.1/1,060') and returns to Coit Road (12.3/960'). Turn left to return to Coyote Creek Trailhead (12.4/940').

Giving Back

The **Pine Ridge Association** assists park staff in designing interpretive materials and presenting educational programs to the public. It offers a volunteer training program. Contact the association or learn more at (408) 779-2728 or **www.coepark.org.**

27 Henry W. Coe State Park:
WILSON PEAK AND VICINITY LOOP

RATINGS	Scenery **7** Difficulty **7** Solitude **9**
ROUND-TRIP DISTANCE	9.4 miles
ELEVATION GAIN/LOSS	+2,500'/–2,500'
RECOMMENDED MAP	*Henry W. Coe State Park Trail and Camping Map* by the Pine Ridge Association
BEST TIMES	March through May
AGENCY	Henry W. Coe State Park, (408) 779-2728, **www.coepark.org**
PERMIT	A first-come, first-served backcountry permit is required. You can self-register at Hunting Hollow Trailhead. Permits are always available.

Highlights

Soaring ridgelines rise above the verdant valley of Hunting Hollow, providing access to the little-traveled southern backcountry of Henry Coe. Remote ponds, inviting woodlands, expansive vistas, ranching history, and the summit of Wilson Peak await.

Hike Overview

The journey makes a counterclockwise loop above and then beyond Hunting Hollow, a linear stream valley along the park's southern boundary. Using a mix of thin single-track paths and wide fire roads, the journey briefly tours Hunting Hollow Creek (fording it several times) before steeply ascending Lyman Wilson Ridge to reach an old ranching field station (Wilson Camp), pleasant Tule and Rodeo ponds, and the 2,651-foot summit of Wilson Peak, the highest in the vicinity. You then cruise high above the park along Steer Ridge before plummeting down the ridge to the trailhead. Expansive and far-reaching views accompany you throughout the journey.

Watch out for periods of heavy rain, when Hunting Hollow Creek can transform from an ankle-deep stream to a thigh-deep muddy torrent. The *Henry W. Coe State Park Trail and Camping Map* is strongly recommended as a complement to the maps in this book. It covers the entire park and all its trails and is available at the park visitor center or can be ordered from the Pine Ridge Association, the park's nonprofit partner (**www.coepark.org**).

Trail Camps

A backcountry permit is required and must be obtained the day of your departure. All permits are first-come, first-served—reservations are *not* accepted—and there is a fee of $5 per night per person. Quotas for each zone are seldom met, and securing a backcountry permit is rarely an issue. Obtain your permit from the self-service station at nearby Hunting Hollow Trailhead (directions below).

This hike travels through the Phegley and Grizzly Gulch backcountry zones, where camping is unrestricted. Campsites are abundant; obtaining water is the challenge. Good options include **Wilson Camp; Rodeo** or **Tule ponds** near the hike's midpoint; or a

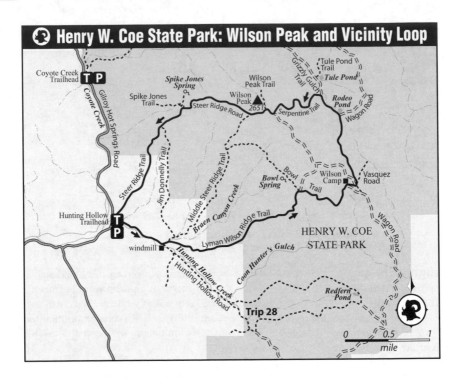

Henry W. Coe State Park: Wilson Peak and Vicinity Loop

small unnamed pond just below **Wilson Peak**. A filter is recommended for treating the often murky pond water. *Camping is prohibited within a half mile of the trailhead.*

Getting There

Take the Leavesley Road exit from Highway 101 in Gilroy and follow Leavesley Road 1.8 miles east to New Avenue. Turn left and follow New Avenue 0.6 mile to Roop Road, and turn right. At this point Roop Road becomes Gilroy Hot Springs Road and reaches Coyote Creek County Park on the left in 3.0 miles. Continue 3.0 miles more past the park entrance to reach Hunting Hollow Trailhead on the right.

Hiking It

Gray pines and sycamores intermingle with coast live oaks and bay

trees around the trailhead parking lot (0.0/860'). Strike out on Hunting Hollow Road, passing a picnic table by the creek and crossing through a gate to immediately make your first ford of Hunting Hollow Creek. Steer Ridge Trail, your return route, awaits on the far side (0.1/860').

Continue on wide, flat Hunting Hollow Road as it heads upstream. Drier blue oak woodland appears immediately to the left, while water-loving sycamores and coast live oaks grow in the moist stream corridor. The road cruises through flat meadows and past sloping woodlands, crossing the creek on four occasions before reaching a pleasant meadow where Lyman Wilson Trail joins on the left (0.7/900').

Let the ascent begin! Bear left on Lyman Wilson Trail, quickly reaching Middle Steer Ridge Trail (0.8/910') at the confluence of Braen Canyon and Hunting Hollow creeks. The route climbs steeply through thick woods, offering intermittent views into Hunting Hollow behind you. The trail ascends along the ridgeline, passes a small brown pond below to the right, and offers increasingly expansive views as it gains elevation.

After a curving switchback, the trail crosses a fence and soon widens. From here, you can see the length of Hunting Hollow. The park's southern border runs along Osos Ridge, hemming Hunting Hollow in to the south. Middle Steer Ridge is immediately west; Steer Ridge—your later destination—rises above it. To the northwest, Coyote Creek cuts a deep canyon on its journey north.

The gradient eventually eases as the route winds high along the grassy ridgeline, even dropping briefly to pass a small pond. The trail next traverses the south side of the ridge, narrowing as it approaches Bowl Trail (2.9/2,150'). Bear right on Bowl Trail to immediately travel above a small pond. You next cross several closely-spaced springs and begin a refreshingly flat traverse with good views of Coon Hunter's Gulch below. Rounding a corner, you drop toward Wilson Camp and by another spring, this one dribbling into a black Rubbermaid tub. Wilson Camp (3.9/2,040') is just ahead.

An old ranch field station, Wilson Camp lies in disrepair; old plumbing, sinks, and other debris lie scattered near the locked building. A designated camping area is located a short distance uphill from the building. Wilson Camp Spring—one of the park's most reliable—emerges from an adjacent faucet.

From camp, follow the wide road uphill to reach a substantial five-way

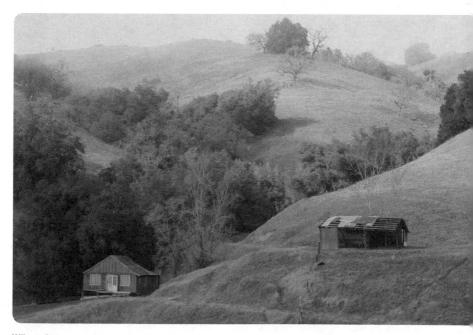

Wilson Camp

junction (4.1/2,140'). From here, you have several options. The shortest variation skips Rodeo and Tule ponds and follows Steer Ridge Road directly to Wilson Peak. The open and exposed ridge walk offers expansive views of hillsides dotted with crusty, elegant blue oaks and reaches the junction with Serpentine Trail in 1.4 miles.

The recommended route (0.9 mile longer) continues north on wide Wagon Road as it traverses upward, then cruises gently downhill along shadier slopes of mixed oak woodlands. It abruptly emerges at a broad, flat divide; Rodeo Pond is a short distance ahead (4.9/2,070'). The pond reflects the mature oak savanna surrounding it and is lively with birds and aquatic life,

especially frogs. Camping options are abundant and nearby hillsides beckon to be explored.

Continuing past the pond, you reach Grizzly Gulch Trail just below the dam. Go straight on Grizzly Gulch Trail, passing through blue oak woodlands en route to the junction with Serpentine Trail on the left (5.3/2,030'). Your continuing route bears left on Serpentine Trail, but take the time to visit nearby Tule Pond, 0.2 mile ahead on Wagon Road. Nice campsites, mature blue oaks, and wispy gray pines highlight this pleasant destination.

Head up Serpentine Trail to immediately begin climbing the single-track path. You rise steadily, passing through broad meadows to ultimately crest at

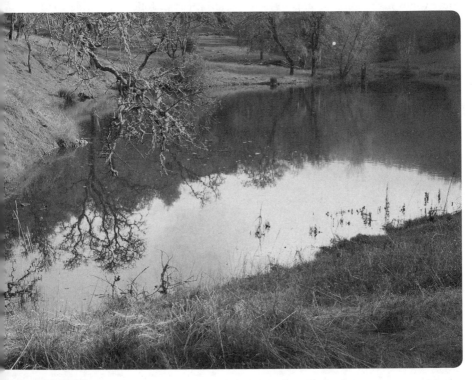

Tule Pond

2,600 feet and meet Steer Ridge Trail (6.2/2,610'). Bear right on the wide road, noting the numerous serpentine outcrops—California's state rock—alongside the trail. Recognize it by its pale, gray-green coloration and waxy, slippery texture.

You then reach Wilson Peak Trail (6.4/2,610'). To make the quick detour to Wilson Peak (2,651'), follow Wilson Peak Trail a few hundred yards to the high point of the rounded summit, indicated by two USGS markers. Views sweep in all directions, including the hills of the little traveled southeast corner of the park. Ample (waterless) campsites can be found in the area, though there is limited shelter from wind; drop off the ridgeline to the north to find some protection.

Continuing on Steer Ridge Trail, you cruise along a grassy, oak-studded ridge with excellent views east and west. To the south, you can spot the distant Santa Lucia Mountains of the Big Sur region.

You next reach Middle Steer Ridge Trail on the left (6.6/2,570'). From here a small pond is visible below Wilson Peak to the north, where a few potential campsites can be found near water.

Remain on Steer Ridge Trail, soon passing another small pond below to your left. Views north stretch all the way to Pine Ridge and the park's main entrance area; ponderosa pines are discernible along the ridgeline. Mount Hamilton Observatory rises beyond. The route gently drops, passes a pond access trail, and then briefly climbs. Enjoy views west into the Coyote Creek

drainage that defines the west-central portion of the park. Views expand as you approach the end of the ridge, overlooking Hunting Hollow and Coyote Creek drainages.

Continue straight on Steer Ridge Road at the junction for Spike Jones Trail—and a nearby unreliable spring—on the right (7.5/2,390'). The road diminishes into grassy paths as you pass Jim Donnelly Trail on the left (7.9/2,170') and enjoy good vantages south—views extend to the peaks of the Monterey Peninsula and adjacent Gabilan Range inland.

The plummet home soon begins. The initial descent is one of easy cruising followed by sharp descents. You then make a direct and radical descent without break, finally ending in a nice shady grove of coast live oaks. The trail continues its descent toward the trailhead—steady but not as severe as before—and passes through nice meadows with views of Coyote Creek. Then the final relentless drop begins, descending rapidly to make a final curving switchback left near the bottom. A steep traversing zigzag finally deposits you on the valley floor (9.3/860'). Hunting Hollow Road and the trailhead are immediately ahead to your right (9.4/860').

Giving Back

The **Pine Ridge Association** assists park staff in designing interpretive materials and presenting educational programs to the public. It offers a volunteer training program. Contact the association or learn more at (408) 779-2728 or **www.coepark.org**.

28 Henry W. Coe State Park:
REDFERN POND

RATINGS	Scenery **7** Difficulty **6** Solitude **8**
ROUND-TRIP DISTANCE	7.6 miles
ELEVATION GAIN/LOSS	+1,500'/–1,500'
RECOMMENDED MAP	*Henry W. Coe State Park Trail and Camping Map* by the Pine Ridge Association
BEST TIMES	March through May
AGENCY	Henry W. Coe State Park, (408) 779-2728, **www.coepark.org**
PERMIT	A first-come, first-served backcountry permit is required. You can self-register at Hunting Hollow Trailhead. Permits are always available.

Highlights

Follow the mellifluous stream of Hunting Hollow to dramatic single-track paths that ascend steep ridgelines to reach tranquil Redfern Pond, the largest in Coe's southern backcountry.

Hike Overview

The journey follows wide, flat Hunting Hollow Road upstream, crossing the waterway at seven different locations. (Watch out for periods of heavy rain, when Hunting Hollow Creek can transform from an ankle-deep stream to a thigh-deep muddy torrent.) It then makes a ridgeline loop to Redfern Pond via single-track Redfern and Phegley Ridge trails, returning back along Hunting Hollow Road. Even with its 1,500-foot elevation gain, the trip is one of the gentler backcountry excursions in this rugged, hilly park. The *Henry W. Coe State Park Trail and Camping Map* is strongly recommended as a complement to the maps in this book. It covers the entire park and all its trails and is available at the park visitor center or can be ordered from the Pine Ridge Association, the park's nonprofit partner (**www.coepark.org**).

Trail Camps

A backcountry permit is required and must be obtained the day of your departure. All permits are first-come, first-served—reservations are *not* accepted—and there is a fee of $5 per night per person. Quotas for each zone are seldom met, and securing a backcountry permit is rarely an issue. Obtain your permit from the self-service station at nearby Hunting Hollow Trailhead (directions below).

This hike travels entirely within the Phegley backcountry zone, where camping is unrestricted. Campsites are abundant; obtaining water is the challenge. Good camping options include **Redfern Pond** at the hike's midpoint, or closer to the trailhead **along Hunting Hollow Creek**. A filter is recommended for Redfern Pond. *Camping is prohibited within a half mile of the trailhead.*

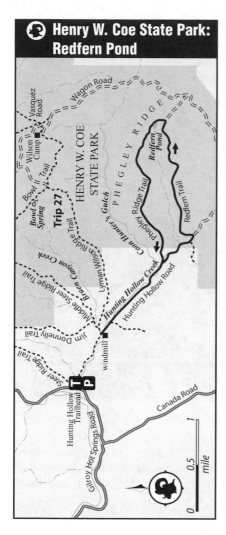

⊘ Henry W. Coe State Park: Redfern Pond

Getting There

Take the Leavesley Road exit from Highway 101 in Gilroy and follow Leavesley Road 1.8 miles east to New Avenue. Turn left and follow New Avenue 0.6 mile to Roop Road, and turn right. At this point Roop Road becomes Gilroy Hot Springs Road and reaches Coyote Creek County Park on the left in 3.0 miles. Continue 3.0 miles more past the park entrance to

reach Hunting Hollow Trailhead on the right.

Hiking It

Gray pines and sycamores intermingle with coast live oaks and bay trees around the trailhead parking lot (0.0/860'). Strike out on Hunting Hollow Road, passing a picnic table by the creek and crossing through a gate to immediately make your first ford of Hunting Hollow Creek. Steer Ridge Trail awaits on the far side (0.1/860').

Continue on wide, flat Hunting Hollow Road as it heads upstream. Drier blue oak woodland appears immediately to the left, while water-loving sycamores and coast live oaks grow in the moist stream corridor. The road cruises easily through flat meadows and past sloping woodlands, crossing the creek on four occasions before reaching a nice meadow and the junction with Lyman Wilson Trail on the left (0.7/900').

Cross the creek again to find a semideveloped site on the far side. Two picnic tables and an old stone grill, complete with a food locker, sit by the water. An old windmill stands here as well, along with a water tank, trough, corral, and other elements of the area's ranching past.

Continuing upstream, the road curves away from the creek and along the edge of wide verdant meadows punctuated by old, twisting valley oaks. Common chaparral species grow along the drier edge of the road, including coffee berry, coyote brush, and gooseberry. The road slowly gains elevation, meeting the creek once again in the middle of the valley (1.5/960'). From here, an unposted trail climbs a short distance to muddy Fish Pond.

Continue on the main road and cross the creek three more times. (You

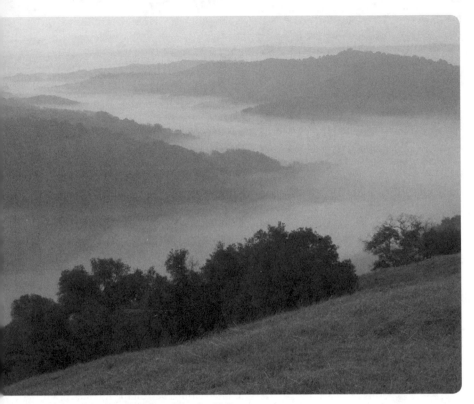

Morning mist fills the valley of Hunting Hollow.

can skip the last two crossings by following a single-track path near the
stream, which rejoins the road at the
confluence of Coon Hunter's Gulch.)
You next pass thin Phegley Ridge
Trail, your return route, on the left
(1.8/980'). The valley palpably narrows as the road crosses the much-
diminished stream four more times and
reaches Redfern Trail (2.3/1,030').

Bear left to head up Redfern Trail,
hopping the creek one last time. The
path is thin, but apparent, a grassy
strip ascending steeply through hillside
meadows. The trail immediately begins
a relentless climb, becoming faint in
places as it closely hews to the ridge-

line. You accelerate high above Hunting Hollow; views east look toward its
headwaters, west toward the trailhead
and Coyote Creek confluence.

The ascent eases slightly as surrounding blue oak woodlands transition to more open valley oak savanna. Nice views west look toward
adjacent Phegley Ridge, your return
route. Looking south, you can pick
out distinctive Fremont Peak and the
mountains of the Monterey peninsula.
You next pass a small chocolate pond
and attain the upper ridge, an open
and exposed section. The ascent soon
resumes, easing somewhat before you
top out and drop briefly to Phegley

Ridge Road (3.8/2,140'). The last few hundred yards of trail are indistinct, marked instead with red and white metal fence posts.

Turn left on Phegley Ridge Road to quickly reach Redfern Pond (3.9/2,100'). Ringed by reeds, the pond sits in a secluded dale surrounded by shady coast live oaks. Potential campsites are abundant. Continue on Phegley Ridge Road, cruising through dense stands of coast live oak. Views eventually open up to the north, revealing adjacent Lyman Wilson Ridge and Steer Ridge beyond it. Wilson Camp can be spotted below, across Coon Hunter's Gulch.

Phegley Ridge Road transitions to an increasingly grassy track as it curves south along the ridgeline and starts a slow descent. The gradient soon steepens, dropping quickly before briefly easing to offer views into Hunting Hollow. Views diminish as the route reenters thick and diverse oak woodlands and narrows to single-track. The forest thickens further as you approach the final plummet, a steep section that drops nearly to the valley floor before easing for the final descent to Hunting Hollow Road (5.8/980'). Bear right and return the way you came to the trailhead (7.6/860').

Giving Back

The **Pine Ridge Association** assists park staff in designing interpretive materials and presenting educational programs to the public. It offers a volunteer training program. Contact the association or learn more at (408) 779-2728 or **www.coepark.org**.

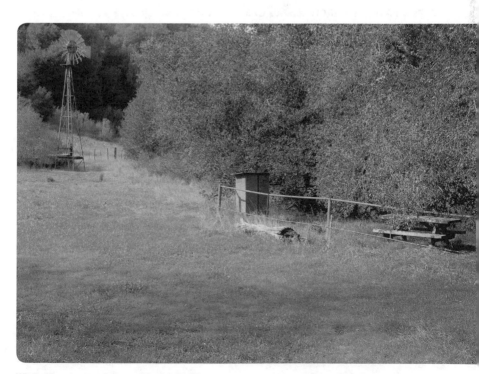

Windmill and campsite near Hunting Hollow

APPENDIX
Bay Area Campgrounds

You don't have to head into the backcountry to experience a blissful night in the Bay Area outdoors. More than two dozen drive-up campgrounds can be found throughout the region in a diverse range of settings and ecosystems, perfect for a quick-and-easy overnight escape. Reservations are necessary for many destinations, especially during the peak summer season. Some locations are open year-round; others close during the off-season. Always check park and campground status before heading out, especially during the winter and spring.

NORTH BAY

Mt. Tamalpais State Park

PANTOLL WALK-IN CAMPGROUND A forested destination in the heart of this rugged and diverse park, Pantoll is a walk-in campground that provides ready access to six nearby trailheads that explore every aspect of the mountain. It's also first-come, first-served, which means that you can secure a site on short notice—provided you arrive sufficiently early. *For more information:* (415) 388-2070, **www.parks.ca.gov**

STEEP RAVINE ENVIRONMENTAL CAMPGROUND Steep Ravine is remote, isolated, and a world away from reality. Ten diminutive cabins and six walk-in campsites perch above breaking waves and rugged cliffs, providing far-reaching views up and down a battered and emergent coastline. With few amenities, abrasive weather, and minimal availability, this is a special place for only the determined few. Reserve far in advance. *Reservations:* (800) 444-7275, **www.reserveamerica.com** *For more information:* (415) 388-2070, **www.parks.ca.gov**

The Marin Headlands

KIRBY COVE CAMPGROUND Kirby Cove is situated at the mouth of a secluded valley immediately west of the Golden Gate Bridge on the shores of the Golden Gate. Accessed via a 0.9-mile one-lane dirt road off-limits to noncampers and inaccessible to RVs and trailers, the campground offers four spacious sites beneath the tall branches of a sheltering forest. Kirby Cove is nearly always full. Reservations are essential. *Reservations:* (800) 365-2267 *For more information:* (415) 331-1540, **www.nps.gov/mahe**

BICENTENNIAL CAMPGROUND This tiny refuge of three tent sites is arranged around a small clearing, and each site accommodates a maximum of only two people. Privacy is minimal but camping here is free. Spectacular views are not available from within the campground itself, but proximity to the many nearby views and attractions make this a worthwhile destination. *For reservations and more information:* (415) 331-1540, **www.nps.gov/mahe**

Samuel P. Taylor State Park

Astride crystalline Lagunitas Creek, shadowed by redwood trees, and surrounded by protected open space, Samuel P. Taylor State Park awaits. Few campgrounds can match its proximity to so many beautiful outdoor destinations. Visitors could easily spend days exploring the vast possibilities of trails and adventures in this park and the surrounding west Marin region. *Reservations:* (800) 444-7275, **www.reserveamerica.com** *For more information:* (415) 488-9897, **www.parks.ca.gov**

China Camp State Park

China Camp State Park tumbles from panoramic ridges to the historic bayshore, delightfully isolated from neighboring San Rafael by intervening topography. Located on the shores of San Pablo Bay, this quiet haven features a mild microclimate that escapes the summer fog and makes it a pleasant camping destination year-round. Add to this its close proximity to San Francisco and Marin County sights and you have a campground ideal for just about everybody. *Reservations:* (800) 444-7275, **www.reserveamerica.com** *For more information:* (415) 456-0766, **www.parks.ca.gov**

Bothe-Napa Valley State Park

Tucked against the western edge of upper Napa Valley, secluded Bothe–Napa Valley State Park provides relief from the area's endless flow of vineyards, traffic, and tourist activity. The only public campground in the area, Bothe (pronounced BO-thee)–Napa makes an ideal base camp for exploring the diverse woodlands of the surrounding hills, marveling at America's largest wooden waterwheel, and savoring the wines of nearby vintners. *Reservations:* (800) 444-7275, **www.reserve america.com** *For more information:* (707) 942-4575

Sugarloaf Ridge State Park

The southern Mayacamas Mountains divide Napa and Sonoma valleys with a sheltered world of pristine California. A thin strip of asphalt winds upward from Sonoma Valley into the heart of these hills, abandoning civilization as it dead-ends in the campground at isolated Sugarloaf Ridge State Park. *Reservations:* (800) 444-7275, **www.reserveamerica.com** *For more information:* (707) 833-5712, **www.parks.ca.gov**

Austin Creek State Recreation Area

A hidden, wild world lurks in the rumpled Coast Range just north of the Russian River. Within easy striking distance of Santa Rosa and the North Bay, Austin Creek State Recreation Area is accessed via a thrilling, one-lane road that first passes beneath the gigantic old-growth redwoods of Armstrong Redwoods State Reserve before climbing more than 1,000 feet at a 12 percent grade to dead-end atop a ridge with spectacular views, where first-come, first-served Bullfrog Pond campground awaits. *For more information:* (707) 869-2015, **www.parks.ca.gov**

SANTA CRUZ MOUNTAINS

Half Moon Bay State Beach

Stroll from your campsite directly to a sandy beach extending miles in either direction. The energy of crashing waves, the extensive coastal views, and the beauty of the open ocean—these are the reasons to come here. Those looking for an isolated destination away from civilization, however, should head elsewhere. *Reservations:* (800) 444-7275, **www.reserveamerica.com** *For more information:* (650) 726-8819, **www.parks.ca.gov**

Butano State Park

The entire upper drainage of Little Butano Creek flows protected through peaceful Butano State Park. The watershed fills a verdant, redwood-filled canyon between steep ridges nearly a thousand feet high with deep, shady camping seclusion in the northern Santa Cruz Mountains. *Reservations:* (800) 444-7275, **www.reserveamerica.com** *For more information:* (650) 879-2040, **www.parks.ca.gov**

Memorial County Park

A small parcel of redwood paradise, the campground at Memorial County Park is set beneath beautiful old-growth trees, a healthy second-growth forest, and a deeply incised creek canyon. Established to protect more than 200 acres of old-growth redwoods from encroaching lumber interests, Memorial County Park was the first of the San Mateo County Parks, dedicated in 1924. *Reservations:* (650) 363-4021, **www.reservations.eparks.net** *For more information:* (650) 879-0238, **www.co.sanmateo.ca.us/portal/site/parks**

Portola Redwoods State Park

Slicing through the western Santa Cruz Mountains, Pescadero Creek flows through a canyon more than 2,000 feet deep. Portola Redwoods State Park protects a wilderness core of this secluded drainage, offering opportunity to commune—and camp within—a vibrant regenerating redwood forest. *Reservations:* (800) 444-7275, **www.reserveamerica.com** *For more information:* (650) 948-9098, **www.parks.ca.gov**

Big Basin Redwoods State Park

Protecting the largest stand of old-growth redwoods south of Humboldt County, Big Basin Redwoods State Park features a forest world like no other in the Bay Area. The first state park in California—the first park anywhere to protect the magnificent coastal redwoods—Big Basin features four campgrounds (Sempervirens, Blooms Creek, Huckleberry, and Wastahi) and more than 80 miles of trails. Located in the heart of the original park acreage, each campground nestles beneath lush redwood forest and offers convenient access to park trails. Tent cabins are also available to rent from a private concessionaire (800-874-8368). *Reservations:* (800) 444-7275, **www.reserveamerica.com** *For more information:* (831) 338-8860, **www.bigbasin.org**

Sanborn County Park

Mixing a landscape of afternoon recreation with the steep slopes and diverse woods of the eastern Santa Cruz Mountains, Sanborn County Park offers something for everybody. Tendrils of redwood forest trail down damp stream gullies and shelter a delightful campground, a huge grassy field perfect for play extends from forest's edge, and a small RV camping lot is tucked in between. *Reservations:* (408) 355-2201, **www.gooutsideand play.org** *For more information:* (408) 867-9959, **www.sccvote.org/portal/site/parks**

Henry Cowell Redwoods State Park

Draining a huge portion of the southern Santa Cruz Mountains, the San Lorenzo River cuts a narrow gorge 500 feet deep less than 10 miles from downtown Santa Cruz. Lush redwood forest fills this moist and secluded canyon, while a surprising world of gnarled ponderosa pine and chaparral grows on the mostly level plateau above the river canyon. Sheltered in this unusual ecological world, a campground lies adjacent to peaceful redwood forest and a nearby grove of massive old-growth trees. *Reservations:*

(800) 444-7275, **www.reserveamerica.com** *For more information:* (831) 438-2396, **www.parks.ca.gov**

Uvas Canyon County Park

Hidden at road's end on the steep eastern flanks of the Santa Cruz Mountains, Uvas Canyon County Park sits near the headwaters of Uvas Creek in a deep, narrow canyon laced with perennial streams and pattering waterfalls. The canyon slopes exist on a rain shadow's edge and provide habitat for a wide variety of trees and plants, perfect for a full ecological taste of the region. *Reservations:* (408) 355-2201, **www.gooutsideandplay. org** *For more information:* (408) 779-9232, **www.sccvote.org/portal/site/parks**

Mount Madonna County Park

Perched atop a ridge within easy striking distance of Monterey Bay and Santa Clara Valley, Mt. Madonna County Park is a fully developed recreation area where young redwood forest veneers dense campgrounds and house ruins whisper memories a hundred years old. Yurts are available for rental in some camping areas. *Reservations:* (408) 355-2201, **www.gooutsideandplay.org** *For more information:* (408) 842-2341, **www.sccvote.org/portal/site/parks**

EAST OF THE BAY

Mount Diablo State Park

A monolithic mountain with eye-popping views, Mt. Diablo (3,849') towers over the surrounding East Bay landscape and harbors three distinct campgrounds upon its vibrant slopes: Juniper, Live Oak, and Junction. Juniper is situated at an elevation of 3,000 feet—the Bay Area's highest drive-in campground. Views are everywhere, sweeping a remarkable 180-degree vista down Diablo's western flanks. Live Oak is at 1,400 feet in a shady mix of trees and foliage and near the interesting geologic exposures of Rock City. First-come, first-served Junction is located at 2,200 feet beneath a shady canopy of blue oak and gray pine. *Reservations:* (800) 444-7275, **www.reserveamerica.com** *For more information:* (925) 837-6119, **www.parks.ca.gov** or **www.mdia.org**

Anthony Chabot Regional Park

A mere ridge away from East Bay cities, Anthony Chabot (pronounced Shuh-BO) campground shelters beneath a canopy of whispering eucalyptus and offers an easy excursion into a surprisingly secluded natural world. City lights are nicely hidden by intervening topography and convenience to metropolitan areas is the advantage here, making it a popular choice for out-of-town visitors and East Bay residents. *Reservations:* (888) 327-2757, **www.reserveamerica.com** *For more information:* (888) 327-2757, **www.ebparks.org**

Del Valle Regional Park

Softly flowing through a broad valley, the ephemeral streamwater of Arroyo del Valle shimmers through an inviting campground before reaching the waters of Lake Del Valle. Surrounding the lake are nearly 4,000 acres of parkland and outdoor recreation in a land of intense seasonal change: lush rain and baking heat, vibrant greens and tawny browns, pressing crowds and empty trails. Secluded in the hills and removed from suburban sight, the park invites visitors year-round. *Reservations:* (888) 327-2757, **www.reserve america.com** *For more information:* (925) 373-0414, **www.ebparks.org**

Sunol Regional Wilderness

Behind the massif of Mission Peak, hidden from the bustling human landscape of the Bay Area, Sunol exists peacefully on nature's terms, on nature's time. The perennial tumble of Alameda Creek beneath the stalwart arms of sycamores, the cycle of seasons in radiant greens and gentle browns, the patient wheeling of raptors across the sky, the steadfast grip of oaks upon hillsides rounded by time.... sweet Sunol. Experience it from the park's tiny campground on the banks of Alameda Creek. *Reservations:* (888) 327-2757, **www.reserve america.com** *For more information:* (510) 544-3249, **www.ebparks.org**

Joseph D. Grant County Park

Hidden in the swales east of San Jose are grassy fields of oaken delight, a quiet world nestled in the foothills of the Bay Area's highest mountains. Largest of the Santa Clara County Parks at nearly 10,000 acres, Joseph D. Grant County Park lies in an isolated valley on a seldom-traveled road and protects a swath of oak woodlands remarkable for its seclusion. *Reservations:* (408) 355-2201, **www.gooutsideandplay.org** *For more information:* (408) 274-6121, **www.sccvote.org/portal/site/parks**

Henry W. Coe State Park

In the heart of the Diablo Range lies a park vast and beautiful, creased with ridges, sliced by canyons, and infused with an incredible variety of life. With 87,000 acres, 700 plants species, 137 bird species, and a lifetime of trails and adventure, Henry W. Coe State Park beckons. Base your adventure from the park's small campground high on ponderosa-studded Pine Ridge. *Reservations:* (800) 444-7275, **www.reserveamerica.com** *For more information:* (408) 779-2728, **www.coepark.org**

Coyote Lake County Park

Filling an oak-studded valley with the dammed waters of Coyote Creek, 635-acre Coyote Lake is a secluded world on the edge of the greater Bay Area. The park is small, the campground closely packed, and swimming or wading in the lake is not permitted. However those in search of fishing, boating, waterskiing, or questing into the southern wilds of Henry W. Coe State Park will find this a pleasant destination. *Reservations:* (408) 355-2201, **www.gooutsideandplay.org** *For more information:* (408) 842-7800, **www.sccvote.org/portal/site/parks**

SELECTED SOURCES AND RECOMMENDED READING

ATLASES

Benchmark California Road and Recreation Atlas. 6th ed. Medford, OR: Benchmark Maps, 2009.

California Atlas and Gazeteer. 1st ed. Yarmouth, ME: DeLorme, 2008.

REGIONAL MAPS

These individual park maps are referenced in the descriptions.

Olmsted, Gerald. A Rambler's Guide to the Trails of the East Bay Hills: Central Section. 3rd ed. Berkeley, CA: The Olmsted and Bros. Map Co., 1995.

———. A Rambler's Guide to the Trails of the East Bay Hills: Northern Section. 3rd ed. Berkeley, CA: The Olmsted and Bros. Map Co., 1995.

———. A Rambler's Guide to the Trails of Mt. Tamalpais and the Marin Headlands. 8th ed. Berkeley, CA: The Olmsted and Bros. Map Co., 1998.

Central San Francisco Peninsula Trails. 2nd ed. Berkeley, CA: Wilderness Press, 2005.

San Francisco Peninsula Parklands Map. Berkeley, CA: Wilderness Press, 2005.

Santa Cruz Mountains Trail Maps 1 and 2. Los Altos, CA: Sempervirens Fund, 1999.

Trail Map of the Southern Peninsula. Palo Alto, CA: The Trail Center, 1999.

FLORA AND FAUNA

Evarts, John, and Marjorie Popper, eds. Coast Redwood: A Natural and Cultural History. Los Olivos, CA: Cachuma Press, 2001.

Fisher, Chris, and Joseph Morlan. Birds of San Francisco and the Bay Area. Redmond, WA: Lone Pine Publishing, 1996.

Johnson, Sharon G., Pamela C. Muick, Bruce M. Pavlik, and Marjorie Popper. Oaks of California. Los Olivos, CA: Cachuma Press, 1991.

Johnston, Verna R. California Forests and Woodlands. Berkeley, CA: University of California Press, 1994.

Keator, Glenn, Ruth M. Heady, and Valerie R. Winemiller. Pacific Coast Fern Finder. Berkeley, CA: Nature Study Guild, 1981.

Lanner, Ronald M. Conifers of California. Los Olivos, CA: Cachuma Press, 1999.

Lederer, Roger. *Pacific Coast Bird Finder*. Berkeley, CA: Nature Study Guild, 1977.

Little, Elbert L. *National Audubon Society Field Guide to North American Trees, Western Region*. New York: Alfred A. Knopf, 1998.

Lyons, Kathleen, and Mary Beth Cooney-Lazaneo. *Plants of the Coast Redwood Region*. Boulder Creek, CA: Looking Press, 1988.

McMinn, Howard, and Evelyn Maino. *An Illustrated Manual of Pacific Coast Trees*. 3rd ed. Berkeley, CA: University of California Press, 2009.

Peterson, Roger Tory. *Western Birds*. 3rd ed. New York: Houghton Mifflin, 1998.

Sims, Lee. *Shrubs of Henry W. Coe State Park*. 2nd ed. Morgan Hill, CA: Pine Ridge Association, 1997.

Spellenberg, Richard. *National Audubon Society Field Guide to North American Wildflowers, Western Region*. New York: Alfred A. Knopf, 1998.

Stuart, John, and John Sawyer. *Trees and Shrubs of California*. Berkeley, CA: University of California Press, 2001.

Watts, Phoebe. *Redwood Region Flower Finder*. Berkeley, CA: Nature Study Guild, 1979.

Watts, Tom. *Pacific Coast Tree Finder*. Berkeley, CA: Nature Study Guild, 1973.

GEOLOGY

Alt, David D., and Donald W. Hyndman. *Roadside Geology of Northern California*. 2nd ed. Missoula, MT: Mountain Press Publishing Company, 2000.

Galloway, Alan J. *Geology of the Point Reyes Peninsula*. Bulletin 202, California Division of Mines and Geology, 1977.

Harden, Deborah R. *California Geology*. 2nd ed. New Jersey: Prentice-Hall, 2003.

Konigsmark, Ted. *Geologic Trips: San Francisco and the Bay Area*. Gualala, CA: GeoPress, 1998.

McPhee, John. *Assembling California*. New York: Farrar, Straus and Giroux, 1993.

USGS. *Geologic Map of California*. 1:750,000. 2010.

Wahrhaftig, Clyde. *A Streetcar to Subduction and Other Plate Tectonic Trips by Public Transport in San Francisco*. Revised ed. Washington, D.C.: American Geophysical Union, 1984.

REGIONAL INFORMATION

California Coastal Resource Guide. California Coastal Commission and Berkeley, CA: University of California Press, 1987.

California Coastal Access Guide. 6th ed. California Coastal Commission and Berkeley, CA: University of California Press, 2003.

Arnot, Phil. *Point Reyes: Secret Places and Magic Moments.* San Carlos, CA: Wide World Publishing/Tetra, 1992.

Briggs, Winslow. *The Trails of Henry W. Coe State Park: Coe Ranch Section.* Morgan Hill, CA: Pine Ridge Association, 2000.

Browning, Peter, ed. *The Discovery of San Francisco Bay: The Portola Expedition of 1769–1770.* Lafayette, CA: Great West Books, 1992.

Cassady, Stephen. *Spanning the Gate.* Santa Rosa, CA: Squarebooks, 1993.

Dunham, Tacy. *Marin Headlands Trail Guide.* Novato, CA: Cottonwood Press, 1989.

Evens, Jules. *Natural History of the Point Reyes Peninsula.* Berkeley, CA: University of California Press, 2008.

Gilliam, Harold, and Ann Lawrence. *Marin Headlands: Portals of Time.* San Francisco, CA: Golden Gate National Park Conservancy, 1993.

Lage, Jessica. *Point Reyes: The Complete Guide to the National Seashore and Surrounding Area.* 1st ed. Berkeley, CA: Wilderness Press, 2004.

Lorentzen, Bob, and Richard Nichols. *Hiking the California Coastal Trail: Volume 1.* 2nd ed. Mendocino, CA: Bored Feet Publications, 2003.

Lowry, Alexander, and Denzil Verardo. *Big Basin.* Los Altos, CA: Sempervirens Fund, 1973.

Margolin, Malcolm. *The East Bay Out.* Revised ed. Berkeley, CA: Heyday Books, 1988.

———. *The Ohlone Way: Indian Life in the San Francisco–Monterey Bay Area.* Berkeley, CA: Heyday Books, 1978.

Okamoto, Ariel Rubissow. *Golden Gate National Parks: Guide to the Parks.* 2nd ed. San Francisco, CA: Golden Gate National Parks Conservancy, 2004.

Paddison, Joshua. *A World Transformed: Firsthand Accounts of California Before the Gold Rush.* Berkeley, CA: Heyday Books, 1999.

Rusmore, Jean. *Bay Area Ridge Trail: The Official Guide for Hikers, Mountain Bikers, and Equestrians.* Berkeley, CA: Wilderness Press, 2008.

Rusmore, Jean, Betsy Crowder, and Frances Spangle. *South Bay Trails: Outdoor Adventures in and Around Santa Clara Valley.* 3rd ed. Berkeley, CA: Wilderness Press, 2001.

————. *Peninsula Trails: Outdoor Adventures on the San Francisco Peninsula.* 4th ed. Berkeley, CA: Wilderness Press, 2004.

Sprout, Jerry, and Janine Sprout. *Golden Gate Trailblazer: Where to Hike, Walk, and Bike in San Francisco and Marin.* 2nd ed. Berkeley, CA: Wilderness Press, 2004.

Taber, Tom. *The Santa Cruz Mountains Trail Book.* 10th ed. San Mateo, CA: The Oak Valley Press, 2006.

Vanderwerf, Barbara. *The Coastside Trail Guidebook.* El Granada, CA: Gum Tree Lane Books, 1995.

Weintraub, David. *East Bay Trails: Outdoor Adventures in Alameda and Contra Costa County.* 2nd ed. Berkeley, CA: Wilderness Press, 2005.

————. *North Bay Trails: Outdoor Adventures in Marin, Napa, and Sonoma Counties.* 2nd ed. Berkeley, CA: Wilderness Press, 2004.

————. *Monterey Bay Trails: Outdoor Adventures in Monterey, Santa Cruz, and San Benito Counties.* Berkeley, CA: Wilderness Press, 2001.

White, Peter. *The Farallon Islands, Sentinels of the Golden Gate.* San Francisco, CA: Scottwall Associates, 1995.

Yaryan, Willie, and Denzil and Jennie Verardo. *The Sempervirens Story: A Century of Preserving California's Ancient Redwood Forest.* Los Altos, CA: Sempervirens Fund, 2000.

Index

About the Author

Matt Heid is the author of *101 Hikes in Northern California* and *Best Backpacking Trips in New England*, a contributor to *Backpacking California*, and a researcher and writer for three Let's Go guides. He holds a degree in earth and planetary science from Harvard University and stays busy pursuing a passion for outdoor writing and remote wilderness adventure in Northern California, Alaska, and New England. He currently lives in Framingham, Massachusetts.

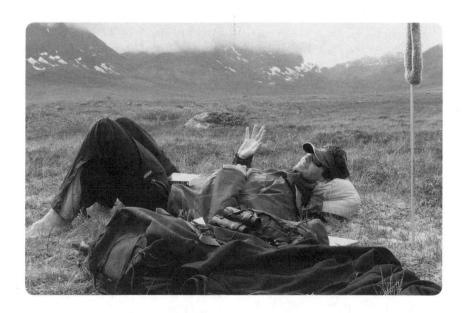